SANTA MONICA COLLEGE LIBRARY

3 5046 00122 7471

W9-CSY-649

NEW OPTIONS FOR
Fertility

NEW OPTIONS FOR
Fertility

A Guide to

In Vitro Fertilization and

Other Assisted Reproduction Methods

SANTA MONICA COLLEGE LIBRARY
SANTA MONICA, CALIFORNIA

Arthur L. Wisot, M.D., and David R. Meldrum, M.D.

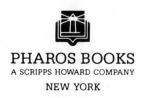

PHAROS BOOKS
A SCRIPPS HOWARD COMPANY
NEW YORK

Copyright © 1990 by Arthur L. Wisot, M.D., Inc., and David R. Meldrum, M.D.

All rights reserved. No part of this book may be reproduced in any form or by any means without written permission of the publisher.

First published in 1990.

Library of Congress Cataloging-in-Publication Data

Wisot, Arthur L.
    New options for fertility: a guide to IVF and other assisted
reproduction methods / by Arthur L. Wisot and David R. Meldrum.
        p.   cm.
    Includes bibliographical references.
    ISBN 0-88687-477-7 : $17.95
    1. Fertilization in vitro. Human—Popular works.   2. Human
reproductive technology—Popular works.   I. Meldrum. David R.
    II.   Title.
    RG135.W57   1990
    618.1'7805—dc20   89-78434
                                                                          CIP

Acknowledgment is made for permission to include previously published material:
Fleming, Anne Taylor, "The Infertile Sisterhood: When the Last Hope Fails." Copyright © 1989 by
The New York Times Company. Reprinted by permission.

Interior design: Bea Jackson
Jacket design and photography: Bea Jackson

Printed in the United States of America

Pharos Books
A Scripps Howard Company
200 Park Avenue
New York, NY 10166

10 9 8 7 6 5 4 3 2 1

This book is dedicated to the ideal of the family—including our own, who make it all worthwhile: Phyllis, David, Andrew, and Jeffrey Wisot and Claudia, Erik, Tiffany, Nicole, and Bret Meldrum.

And to parents—including our own, whose love and support made it all possible: Hilly and Helen Wisot and Roy and Margaret Meldrum.

ACKNOWLEDGMENTS

Our deep appreciation goes to our editor, Hana Lane, and our publisher, David Hendin, whose foresight was instrumental in the publication of this book; our literary agent and adviser, Les Lang, whose support and advice has contributed enormously to the project; Dr. Gene Naftulin for his contributions in the field of male infertility; Georgia and Nat Kramer for their legal counsel; Claudia Meldrum for her support and sharing her own personal struggle with infertility; and Phyllis Wisot for her editing, which greatly improved the original manuscript, and her tireless preparation of the appendices.

Our heartfelt thanks go to the members of the AMI-South Bay Hospital IVF team, our office staffs, and others whose critical reading of portions of the manuscript and ideas were vital: Minda Hamilton; Bivian Marr, RN, RNP; Cathy Stubbs, RN; Willetta Allen; Cathy Bradley; Chris Puanglarplai; Gayle Killen, RN, CNP; Deborah Clark; Victoria Scogins; Yvette Barnett and Barbara Lang.

We especially appreciate the contribution of all our patients, many of whom offered suggestions and are anonymously represented in the book. However, certain individuals generously offered to share their stories publicly so that others may benefit from their experiences: Cheryl and Jeff Scruggs, Patty and Brad Woods, Jane and Terry Mohr, Nancy and Dick Woodka, and Penny and Roger Berry.

We would also like to thank Leslie Nies and her staff at Serono Symposia, USA (Serono Laboratories, Inc.), for permission to use their medical illustrations.

We could not have completed this project without the love and constant support of our families—Phyllis, David, Andrew, and Jeff Wisot, Helen Wisot, Richard and Elaine Wisot, Bob and Judie Friedlander, Ann and Irving Bernstein, and Claudia, Erik, Tiffany, Nicole, and Bret Meldrum.

Contents

Introduction

You do become desperate. You go through periods where you cry for no reason and you want someone to help you. If someone says they can help you, if they say stand on your head after sex you will try that. If your friends say, gee, I held a chicken foot up and it worked for me you will try that. If a man says, thousands and thousands of dollars, if you can afford it you will try it.

Actress Jo Beth Williams,
testifying before the congressional
subcommittee's hearing on Consumer
Protection Issues Involving In Vitro
Fertilization Clinics, March 9, 1989

This statement from a person who has struggled with an infertility problem is not unusual. Also not unusual is the difficulty infertile couples have in obtaining valid information regarding the high-tech procedures that have become dispassionately known as assisted reproductive technology (ART). These couples are so desperate, the technology is so complex, and the means of gauging success are so confusing that, as Dr. Alan deCherney of Yale testified at the hearing, "infertility patients are exceptionally vulnerable to exploitation." Subcommittee chairman Rep. Ron Wyden (D-Ore.) agreed, concluding that "infertile couples find it extremely difficult to obtain clear, understandable and unbiased information about the performance of IVF clinics. Many of these couples are desperate to have children. They have been on an emotional roller coaster for years, attempting to conceive through a variety of procedures. They are vulnerable to exploitation."

That potential for exploitation is manifest in a host of claims from centers throughout the country regarding their success rates. Consider these examples:

• An ad in the Chicago *Tribune* in July 1988 stated that a particular clinic reports a confirmed pregnancy rate of 30 percent, but they don't say 30 percent of what. We are not told whether this is 30 percent of

all patients starting, those who went through only part of the program,
only those who completed the program, or a particular select group of
patients. Stating a percentage is meaningless without defining the group
being measured.

• The September 1988 issue of *Better Homes & Gardens* featured an
attractive advertisement including pictures of babies and the claim that
"four of the first twelve patients have achieved a pregnancy.... Our
first test tube baby is due this October.... Our success rate is an
impressive 30 percent, well above the national average." But what does
success mean? Presumably the 30 percent refers to four of the first
twelve patients who became pregnant. However, no babies had been
born yet, and the number of cycles was so small as to be almost
meaningless.

In December 1988, the ad ran again, but without the "Our success
rate is an impressive 30 percent, well above the national average."
Why was this sentence deleted? In reviewing the data presented to the
subcommittee from this clinic it appeared that four of the first twenty
got pregnant. That would mean that after the first twelve patients, no
pregnancies were achieved. Yet the ad continued to state that the first
four of twelve got pregnant. Actually, this clinic formally reported a
live birth and continuing pregnancy rate of 11 percent per cycle
stimulated by fertility drugs and 13 percent per cycle resulting in eggs
being retrieved.

• In September 1988, IVF Australia ran an ad in the Boston *Globe*
stating that 236 babies had been born as the result of IVF Australia
programs. That figure is correct. However, IVF Australia has two
programs in the U.S.—and that ad ran when the Boston program was
only three months old. Exactly the same techniques were being used by
the newer program and the same rate of success was naturally
expected, but the consumer was not made aware that the Boston
program was relatively new.

• An ad described by syndicated columnist Ellen Goodman included a
picture of a newborn with the headline BEFORE YOU LET GO OF THE DREAM,
TALK TO US. The text described "There's no other perfume like it, the
smell of a newborn: a milk-scent, warm scent, cuddle essence. Her skin
a new kind of velvet. Toes more wrinkled than cabbage, yet roselike.
Tender, soft, totally trusting; a blessing of your own.... That dream
might still come true for you. New techniques can resolve many

infertility problems, including some that were previously considered hopeless." Now, this may all be true, but Goodman concluded that such ads play upon the vulnerabilities of the infertile couple. They certainly do not provide important information about the chance of becoming pregnant.

Advertising claims are not limited to IVF programs, but also include devices intended to improve fertility. An ad for a basal body temperature device called Rabbit, for instance, proclaimed: " 'Yes! You Will Become Pregnant' if you use Rabbit." In small type underneath is the disclaimer "and you're medically able to conceive."

Even quoted statistics are often misleading or downright inaccurate. Some programs quote national figures. Others present the statistics in a favorable light. For example, they may cite a time interval when they did exceptionally well and quote a success rate that does not reflect their overall experience. Except for the subcommittee report, statistics on individual centers have not been released to the public. Figures on 155 programs are currently being collected by the Society for Assisted Reproductive Technology (SART) but are published in a medical journal as pooled statistics. So the most anyone can learn is the average experience across the country, not the rates for specific programs.

The scope of the problem is large since IVF clinics are a tremendous growth industry. The government's Office of Technology Assessment estimates that more than a billion dollars was spent in 1987 on infertility treatment for the approximately 2.4 million couples experiencing the problem. They estimated that $30 to $40 million were spent on IVF procedures alone. Also, the number of patients undergoing treatment is increasing. Treatment cycles reported to the congressional survey increased from 8167 in 1987 to 10,105 in 1988.

These procedures are being performed in a variety of settings, from university centers to single-doctor offices. There is a wide spectrum of qualifications—some of these practitioners have inadequate training or experience. At present there is no professional or government oversight of this industry. Any physician can hold himself out as a fertility specialist. Embryo laboratories are not subject to the most cursory inspections required of other labs.

Yet, despite all these vital consumer issues, the technology can be successful. Some of the best programs are now legitimately reporting that 20 percent to 25 percent of their patients take home a baby for each patient having an egg retrieval procedure. It is the prospective user of this technology who has the job of seeking information and finding those clinics that are achieving the best results. Jo Beth Williams, who played the surrogate birthmother Mary Beth Whitehead in the TV movie *Baby M.*, concluded her testimony to the subcommittee "We, the infertile couples, need to learn what questions to ask. We need to know where we can get the right answers."

ABOUT THE AUTHORS

Co-author Dr. Arthur Wisot developed his interest in infertility as a resident physician in obstetrics and gynecology at the Long Island Jewish Medical Center in New Hyde Park, New York. As he worked in the various disciplines included in obstetrics and gynecology, he developed an affinity to the patients who were having trouble conceiving. Although infertility treatments were in their infancy, he could sense the importance to the patients of overcoming their infertility problem.

His interest in infertility expanded during continuing education courses in all the new developments, including special training in microsurgery. He was instrumental in the development of the In Vitro Fertilization Center at AMI-South Bay Hospital in Redondo Beach, California, in conjunction with Dr. Meldrum. In addition to helping Dr. Meldrum develop the center, Dr. Wisot learned all of the clinical monitoring protocols and procedures so that he now works alongside Dr. Meldrum in one of the most successful in vitro fertilization (IVF) programs in the nation.

In addition to his clinical interest in infertility and assisted reproduction, Dr. Wisot has long been involved in consumer issues relating to health care issues. He has worked to inform the public about these issues in many newspaper and magazine articles and as the consumer-health reporter for KHJ-TV, Channel 9, in Los Angeles. This media experience led to his serving as host and medical editor of "Physicians' Journal Update" and "Obstetrics and Gynecology Update" on Lifetime Medical Television, informing physicians on new medical and surgical developments. In addition, he is associate clinical professor in the Department of Obstetrics and Gynecology at the UCLA School of Medicine.

Co-author Dr. David Meldrum's interest in infertility began in a personal circumstance. When he became engaged to his wife Claudia, she informed him that she might not be able to have children and indicated that she would understand if he wanted to break off the engagement because of this possibility. Childlessness would be devastating to her, so she felt that he should be aware of this possibility. Although her desire to have a family was not all-consuming, her main goal in life at that time was to be a good wife and mother. But her fiancé realized that her problem (lack of ovulation) could probably be solved through drugs then available. Although the treatments could be difficult, he was relatively certain, as a young intern, that if they persevered they would be successful.

By this time (1973) David Meldrum had already decided to go into obstetrics and gynecology, but their own difficulty moved him in the direction of caring for patients with infertility. Claudia was initially given the drug clomiphene to try to stimulate ovulation. She showed signs of responding but apparently did not ovulate despite increasing doses. (A yet-to-be-discovered advance in the treatment of ovulatory problems—the combination of a simple injection of HCG with clomiphene—might have worked for her.)

After three failed cycles on clomiphene, Claudia and David made the decision to go on to treatment with hMG, a powerful naturally occurring hormone designed to stimulate the ovaries. A natural product, it is very expensive, requires daily injections, and holds an increased risk of multiple births. We now have sophisticated ways of monitoring patients using this medication, such as observing estrogen levels and ultrasound examinations. But, in those days, doctors monitored patients by following the changes in their cervical mucus, looking for indications that the patient's estrogen level was high.

Claudia went through six cycles of hMG before she finally became pregnant. Despite Dave's optimism, they had also applied for a baby through adoption. During that successful cycle, Claudia was probably overstimulated; that is, she produced too many eggs, increasing the risk of multiple pregnancy. If they were using the methods of monitoring patients we use today, this successful cycle would probably have been bypassed and pregnancy would not have occurred. In addition, this successful cycle happened after she resumed the HMG treatments following six relaxing months in Spain away from infertility treatments.

Claudia feels that their trip minimized the importance of the problem and relieved much of the pressure by some time away from an anxious family.

An ultrasound in early pregnancy revealed the presence of twins. The Meldrums were delighted. By about twenty-six weeks, the ultrasound found a third baby. Triplets! The Meldrums were now getting nervous. The fourth baby was never discovered by the ultrasound. Bret, their fourth child, was a complete surprise to everyone. Claudia delivered prematurely at thirty-four weeks. All four babies were delivered normally and ranged in weight from 2.75 to 3.75 pounds. The birth order was Erik, Tiffany, Nicole, and Bret. Dave describes the experience as overwhelming. Claudia did not know that she had had quads until she had awakened from the emergency general anesthesia she was given because of a prolapsed umbilical cord during the birth of Erik. She had not planned on an anesthetic and was hoping for a natural childbirth using the Lamaze technique. Following the births, the main concern was for the immediate welfare of these four premature babies in the newborn intensive care unit at the UCLA Medical Center. However, the Meldrum quads did very well and came home from the hospital three to five weeks after birth.

The quads were born during Dave's first year on the UCLA faculty. At that point the focus of his practice was infertility, mainly tubal microsurgery. He became interested in IVF as he realized that some patients would be clearly better treated with this new method. This was a natural outgrowth of his belief that the clinician had to find the best treatment for each individual patient. He felt that there should be no need for a patient to go through surgery if IVF could produce the same or better results with less risk.

Infertility was not as great a stress emotionally for Dave and Claudia as for some other couples because they always looked at it as a problem that could be solved. Although she was not as optimistic as Dave, Claudia feels his positive attitude was contagious and was supportive for her. With the advances in infertility treatment and assisted reproduction since that time, he feels that almost every couple can approach the problem with the same sense of confidence they did. He thinks that if couples maintain a sense of optimism that their problem can be solved, there can be less stress associated with infertility. He feels that this is a realistic approach, given today's technology. If a couple perseveres through four cycles of IVF or even egg donation, they will have an excellent chance to have their family. Perhaps this factor is best illustrated by a picture hanging in the IVF Center which was donated by one of our successful couples. It shows two gulls in flight with a quote from Vergil beneath. "They can because they think they can."

Dr. Meldrum learned IVF during a subbatical in Australia in 1982 and set up both the clinical and laboratory aspects of the UCLA IVF program. After twelve years on the full-time faculty he moved the program to South Bay Hospital in 1986.

Over the years Dr. Meldrum has been a pioneer in many of the clinical and laboratory techniques involved in in vitro fertilization. He is a frequent lecturer and has published close to a hundred articles and chapters related to microsurgery, female hormone problems, and assisted reproductive technology. In addition to his position as director of the IVF Center at AMI-South Bay Hospital, he maintains his affiliation with UCLA as a clinical professor in the Department of Obstetrics and Gynecology. He is currently president of the Society of Assisted Reproduction Technology (SART) of the American Fertility Society.

To provide a comprehensive picture of male fertility, Dr. Gene Naftulin helped with the sections relating to male infertility. Dr. Naftulin is a urologist specializing in male infertility, director of the Fatherhood Center at AMI-South Bay Hospital, and assistant clinical professor in the Department of Urology at the UCLA School of Medicine.

WHY WE ARE WRITING THIS BOOK

Both authors believe that not enough information is available to the public regarding assisted reproduction. In addition, there is a great deal of confusion over ethical issues regarding this new technology, and especially about the validity of success rates and the place of these procedures in the treatment plan for infertility. We also strongly feel that most of the information the public receives is not presented in the proper perspective. We are writing this book to help infertile couples become better consumers by providing them with what Jo Beth Williams says they need—the right questions to ask and the means to interpret the answers.

In order to give you enough of an understanding to make the proper interpretations, we review basic reproductive science and describe all the alternatives for maximizing your chances of conception. You cannot understand this advanced technology without knowing the basics of reproduction. We discuss the conditions that cause infertility, how to test for them and conventional fertility treatments because assisted reproduction should not even be considered until conventional treatments have been exhausted. All of the current assisted reproduction techniques are explored in detail and patients' experiences with these procedures are included. We provide criteria for the selection of a program, including detailed information about how success rates are calculated and how they can be compared among programs. We explore special considerations for the prenatal care of an IVF patient who is successful. And in instances when the best medical science has to offer is not enough, we look at the use of donors for sperm and eggs. Finally, we look toward the future, considering both scientific and consumer issues.

The book also contains appendices providing you with the actual facts and figures on all the programs which reported voluntarily to the congressional survey, the names and addresses of those programs, and a glossary of terms and abbreviations, resources for further information. We've also provided twenty questions and answers for the couple who want information at a glance.

HOW TO USE THIS BOOK

For the most detailed information, read the entire book. If you are already very familiar with reproductive anatomy, read those chapters anyway because they will provide a good review. The sections on causes, diagnosis, and conventional treatment will ensure that you have had all the proper tests and treatment before going on to ART (assisted reproductive technology) procedures.

Some may choose to use the book primarily as a reference. If that's your desire, the index will help you find the material you need. In this case, we recommend frequent use of the glossary to help you with abbreviations and terms that may not be totally familiar to you.

THE BOTTOM LINE

This book *can* help you get pregnant! As we will remind you throughout its pages, with persistence and proper choices you can maximize your chance to conceive. Of course, we can't guarantee that you'll succeed, but we can help you find the way to give it your best shot. We sincerely hope that each of you can fulfill your dream of having a baby.

NEW OPTIONS FOR
Fertility

one

Little Miracles

"IT'S A MIRACLE EVERY TIME"

" **I** t's a miracle every time!" said Robert Young as the compassionate, caring Marcus Welby, M.D. just after he had delivered a baby in one of the weekly episodes of that popular television series.

That statement might sound like a cliché coming from the lips of Marcus Welby. But it's true. Once you understand all the complex processes that must occur to conceive and carry a baby to delivery, you will agree that it *is* a miracle every time a healthy baby is born.

The "Little Miracles" we are talking about in this book are the healthy babies conceived through assisted reproductive technology (ART) like Greta, the first baby born in the United States as the result of ultrasound-guided egg retrieval in an IVF procedure. The best-known ART procedures are in vitro fertilization (IVF) and gamete intrafallopian transfer (GIFT). When Greta was born, the use of ultrasound was a new technique to obtain the mother's eggs without surgery and was an important milestone in assisted reproductive technology.

ASSISTED REPRODUCTION

What exactly is "assisted reproduction?" The key word is *assisted*. Actually, any kind of help we give a couple in achieving a pregnancy could be called assisted reproduction, from simply maximizing a couple's chances of achieving a pregnancy by teaching them to properly time intercourse to using the most sophisticated techniques to help a single sperm fertilize an egg in the laboratory.

But the term usually refers to the more sophisticated types of infertility treatments, which can be identified by their acronyms—IVF, GIFT, ZIFT, PROST, TE(S)T—abbreviations that may not have meaning to you yet.

If all of this doesn't sound sexy to you, it isn't! In fact, by the time you are involved in anything to do with assisted reproduction, you are probably living your life around your or your partner's menstrual cycle, taking daily injections, having almost daily ultrasound examinations and blood tests, producing semen on demand in a little room with appropriate reading material, and perhaps even undergoing surgery. Any relationship between sex and reproduction went out the window a long time ago. But, if you want a miracle...

LITTLE MIRACLES

Some would argue that the word *miracle* is overused in our field. But we find it frequently and justifiably applied to the type of work we do because many of the people who benefit from assisted reproduction thought they were *hopelessly* infertile before this technology was developed. When someone is desperate, with no expectation of success, remedy, or cure, and succeeds, you can see how *miracle* readily applies.

We see this hopelessness every day. Patty was a young woman whose pelvic organs were left seriously damaged by infection from a Dalkon Shield IUD. She had suffered through ectopic pregnancies, years of infertility, and even multiple attempts at in vitro fertilization. Having her own baby appeared hopeless. Finally, after her third transfer of frozen embryos, she achieved her dream with the birth of her son, Brian. Just moments after Brian was born, Patty's husband Brad sat at Patty's bedside looking at his son and said with tears of joy in his eyes: "I can't believe it. It's a miracle."

But, do we believe that we are really creating miracles? Of course not! The couples are creating the miracles through modern technology with the *assistance* of a team of professionals. That is why it is termed assisted reproductive technology. In fact, this is one of the few areas in medicine where clinical physicians and scientists, such as embryologists, bring together the clinical art and the science of medicine to benefit patients.

Greta and Brian are symbolic of the little miracles you will be meeting in this book. You will meet many more as you learn about assisted reproduction, but keep in mind that although the babies themselves may be little, the miracle their birth represents is as large as any miracle gets.

A DOZEN YEARS AND FIFTEEN THOUSAND BABIES LATER

Assisted reproductive technology in humans is relatively new. At an international congress in Jerusalem in April 1989, the first decade of in vitro fertilization—fertilization that takes place out of the body—was reviewed. The term *in vitro fertilization* literally means "fertilized in glass" and was first demonstrated with rabbits in 1959 by Dr. M. C. Chang. In fact, much of the technology we now use had first been used by scientists in animal husbandry many years before it was applied to humans. Physicians are relative latecomers to this technology.

The era of assisted reproduction in humans began with attempts at in vitro fertilization by teams in England and Australia about fifteen years ago. These efforts culminated in the first successful birth (Louise Brown) in England in 1978. Drs. Patrick Steptoe and Robert Edwards achieved this milestone by obtaining an egg from the mother's ovary during a natural cycle and then placing the resulting embryo back into the mother's uterus. The first success was followed fairly rapidly by pregnancies in Australia (Royal Women's Hospital, Melbourne) in 1980 and in the United States (Eastern Virginia Medical School, Norfolk) in 1981. As of late 1989 there had been an estimated fifteen thousand births in the world, and what once took years to achieve is now a routine medical treatment. According to a *New York Times* report, France boasts one of the highest success rates with 3600 IVF babies born in 1987. In the United States a total of 5500 IVF babies have been born, as well as 3125 claimed by Australia, 1070 in Asia and Africa, 750 in Israel, and 100 in Japan as of the April 1989 world congress.

In 1984, the first pregnancy as the result of gamete intrafallopian transfer (GIFT) was reported by Dr. Ricardo Asch in San Antonio, Texas. In this procedure, the eggs are retrieved by laparoscopy, a procedure in which a telescopic device is inserted through the navel and the eggs are removed by means of a needle placed through the abdominal wall. These eggs are then placed with sperm directly into the fallopian tubes to allow fertilization to take place in the natural location. Also achieved in 1984 was the first human pregnancy resulting from an egg donated by another woman.

Steptoe and Edwards' first pregnancy and those that followed shortly thereafter were achieved using the woman's natural cycle. The woman was allowed to ovulate normally, her cycle was monitored, and one egg was retrieved before it would normally be released from the ovary. In order to make the process more efficient and successful, before long medication was tried to produce multiple eggs based on the concept that you could improve success rates by implanting more than one embryo. Subsequently, much of the research in IVF has been devoted to finding efficient, yet safe, stimulation regimens.

Another milestone was the discovery in Australia by Dr. Alan Trounson that since the eggs were being retrieved early, before they were ready for fertilization, a period of incubation of the eggs prior to adding the sperm would dramatically increase fertilization and thus pregnancy rates.

While stimulation protocols and fertilization techniques were being refined, the method of obtaining the eggs was undergoing change. At the beginning, laparoscopy was being utilized for all egg retrievals. This meant the patients had to go through outpatient surgery under anesthesia. However, with the development of ultrasound techniques most egg retrievals are now being performed by an ultrasound-guided needle inserted into the ovary through the vagina. This can be done with sedation rather than under anesthesia and is not considered a surgical procedure. In addition, the ultrasound approach can generally be done in less time and has a low complication rate. The first ultrasound retrievals in the world were performed in Sweden by Dr. Mats Wikland and in Denmark by Dr. Susan Lenz. The first ultrasound egg retrieval in the United States resulting in successful pregnancy was Greta, and was performed by Dr. Meldrum's IVF program, then at UCLA.

Greta's parents, Nancy and Dick, are another example of the value of perseverance in achieving success. Their major infertility problem was endometriosis. Nancy was working as a consumer and health reporter with Dr. Wisot at KHJ-TV in Los Angeles at the time she was going through hormonal treatment for her endometriosis with Dr. Meldrum at UCLA. Dick was working as a technical director at neighboring Fox Tape. Nancy not only had major surgery to remove substantial amounts of endometriosis, but also had to undergo hormonal treatments for the endometriosis and an additional operation to correct tubal problems. Still, she did not get pregnant.

She and Dick decided to try the new technique' of IVF and went through an unsuccessful IVF cycle with the eggs retrieved by laparoscopy. At about that time, the first successful egg retrievals using abdominal ultrasound were being reported in Sweden and Denmark. Dr. Meldrum was preparing to use the new technique and Nancy and Dick decided to give it another try. Using ultrasound as a guide, the needle was placed through the bladder into the ovary. Two eggs were retrieved and fertilized and the resulting embryos were placed into her uterus.

Nancy is now pregnant again. But this time she and Dick did it on their own, without IVF. Nancy is one of ten patients we have had with endometriosis who, after IVF pregnancies, have conceived on their own. For decades doctors have believed that pregnancy can improve endometriosis and prevent its recurrence. Nancy and the other nine patients are testimony to the correctness of that belief.

We are now over a dozen years and more than fifteen thousand babies into the era of assisted reproduction. The development of this field has occurred rapidly. But we feel that the clinical methods we now use are unlikely to be dramatically different in the next dozen years. Rather, we are beginning a phase of fine-tuning of laboratory techniques and evolution of preferred methods that will result in consistently good results by many programs.

two

The Female Partner

EAT YOUR VEGETABLES!

At some time or other as children we all had the experience of an adult telling us "Eat your vegetables. They're good for you!" Our advice regarding the information in this chapter is similar: Read this chapter. It's good for you!

Actually, it's essential. A discussion of the normal anatomy and reproductive process in the female is not all that exciting and may not be what you want to read about. But, in order to understand the complexities of the technology we describe later in the book, you will need to know the basics. Believe us! By the way, it's probably a pretty good idea to eat your vegetables too.

ANATOMY

We will be concentrating on the anatomy of two areas of the body—the base of the brain and the pelvis. (See Figure 1)

At the base of the brain lie two important structures, the hypothalamus and the pituitary gland. The hypothalamus regulates many of the cyclic body functions, such as the menstrual cycle. The pituitary gland, often called the master gland of the body, is located near the hypothalamus and receives its instructions from the hypothalamus to perform its many functions.

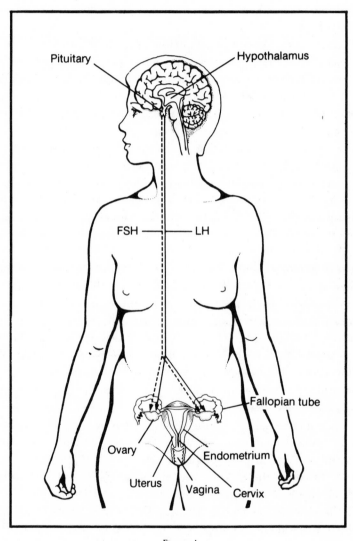

Figure 1

In the pelvis, we are concerned with the female reproductive organs that are responsible for the production and transport of eggs and the carrying of a pregnancy. These include:

- **THE VAGINA**—the canal between the outside and the lower part of the uterus.
- **THE CERVIX**—the lower part of the uterus, which extends into the upper part of the vagina and is the opening into the upper part of the woman's reproductive tract. The cervix is vulnerable to many different types of infection, which can then travel upward into the upper parts of the reproductive system and cause problems with fertility. (Examples of such infections are gonorrhea and chlamydia.)
- **THE UTERUS**—a muscular organ normally the size and shape of a pear. Surrounded by the muscular tissue of the uterus is its lining, the endometrium. This lining fluctuates with the menstrual cycle, preparing itself to receive a pregnancy; and when a pregnancy is not begun in a particular cycle, the lining is broken down and leaves the body as the menstrual flow. The endometrium connects below to the cervix and above to the fallopian tubes.
- **THE FALLOPIAN TUBE**—coming off each side of the top of the uterus, these delicate, thin tubal structures lead from the uterus to the region of the ovaries. Each tube is 10 to 12 centimeters (4 to 5 inches) long. At the end of each tube is a particularly delicate structure called the fimbria. The fimbriae sweep across the ovary to pick up the egg.

  Proper functioning of the tubes is dependent upon all of the microscopic features within it working properly, as even small anatomic alterations can result in tubal malfunctioning. This can lead to a pregnancy getting stuck in a particular portion of the tube, as in an ectopic pregnancy. In other cases, partial or complete obstruction may result in infertility (delay in becoming pregnant) or sterility (permanent inability to get pregnant).
- **THE OVARY**—the ovaries are the female's gonads. Gonads are glands that produce gametes, the basic reproductive germ cells (eggs), in the case of the female partner. The ovaries, oval-shaped organs about 3 centimeters (a little over an inch) in length, are located along each pelvic wall. At the time of a female's birth the ovaries contain all the germ cells (potential eggs) she will need for her lifetime. During fetal life, it is estimated that there are about six million eggs (oocytes)

present in the ovaries. By birth, the number of germ cells has been reduced to approximately one to two million with a further reduction to around 300,000 to 400,000 by puberty. During a woman's reproductive life, she will average about 500 menstrual cycles, utilizing one egg in each of those cycles. So what happens to all the other eggs before she reaches menopause? Some may start to develop, but when one is "chosen" to become the fully developed egg of that cycle, the others degenerate. Some just never develop. It is a system with an incredible amount of reserve, about a thousand to one at puberty—for every egg that develops, a thousand are discarded.

PHYSIOLOGY

Physiology is the study of how the body functions and is really not much more complex than anatomy. Again, we'll break it down into the same two areas of the body we discussed under anatomy.

At the base of the brain: Beginning at puberty, the hypothalamus starts putting out substances to stimulate the pituitary to secrete a number of hormones that, in turn, stimulate the function of other glands in the body—that's why the pituitary is called the master gland. The glands it stimulates that concern us here are the gonads (ovaries). The substances released by the pituitary gland are gonadotropins (hormones that stimulate the gonads). The substance produced by the hypothalamus that causes release of the gonadotropins is called gonadotropin-releasing hormone (GnRH). It makes sense: *Gonadotropin-releasing hormone (GnRH) from the hypothalamus causes the release of gonadotropins from the pituitary gland.*

Two different gonadotropins produced by the pituitary mediate the monthly development of an egg. The egg develops in a structure called a follicle—a fluid-filled area surrounded by supporting cells within which the egg develops. The first gonadotropin that stimulates the growth of the follicle is called follicle-stimulating hormone (FSH). When the egg is ripe and ready to come out of the ovary, a second gonadotropin is produced in a large surge to cause release of the egg (ovulation). This also results in a change of the follicle into a structure (corpus luteum) designed to produce hormones to support implantation of the embryo into the endometrium. This second gonadotropin is

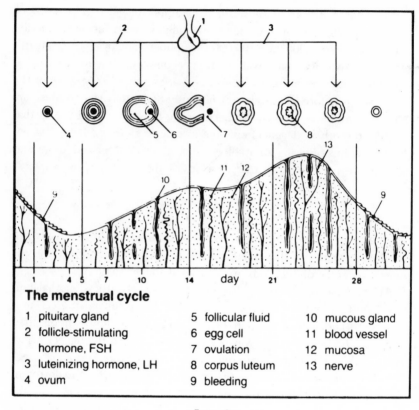

The menstrual cycle

1 pituitary gland	5 follicular fluid	10 mucous gland
2 follicle-stimulating hormone, FSH	6 egg cell	11 blood vessel
	7 ovulation	12 mucosa
3 luteinizing hormone, LH	8 corpus luteum	13 nerve
4 ovum	9 bleeding	

Figure 2

called luteinizing hormone (LH). Actually, LH is produced in small amounts throughout the cycle, but it is this surge of LH we are interested in now.

To review: *The hypothalamus produces GnRH, which stimulates the pituitary to produce FSH and LH. The large pulse of LH triggers ovulation.*

In the pelvis: Meanwhile, in the pelvis three organs respond to these cyclic changes in the gonadotropins. (See Figure 2)

The ovary both responds to the changes in the gonadotropins and mediates the response of the endometrium. Physicians usually count the day a woman starts her menstrual period as Day 1 of the cycle. At about the time of the menstrual period increasing secretion of FSH and small amounts of LH lead to the selection of several eggs to start developing. One of these eggs will eventually become the dominant follicle for that month. Under the stimulation of the FSH and LH, the process of maturation of the egg cell within that follicle begins. In fact, we can now indirectly observe the development of that follicle with ultrasound. We can monitor the increase in size of the follicle, which is a reflection of the accumulation of follicular fluid and maturation of the egg.

The follicle consists of: (1) the egg cell; (2) the shell (zona pellucida); and (3) the corona and cumulus layers surrounding the egg, consisting of granulosa cells that proliferate and produce the hormone estrogen. So another way we can monitor the development of the follicle is by measuring the level of estradiol, one of the estrogens we can measure in the blood. The number of follicles maturing in any one cycle and the degree of maturity reached by these follicles is directly proportional to the amount of FSH and LH present and the sensitivity of the individual's ovary to these gonadotropins. As you might expect, we can cause multiple eggs to develop and mature by giving a woman high doses of gonadotropins.

Of several follicles that begin developing during the menstrual cycle, one will usually progress to maturity by Day 14 in the average woman's cycle. When the follicle reaches maturity, the associated increase of estradiol leads to a surge of LH from the pituitary. This results in the rupture of the follicle and release of the egg (Day 15) and the development of the corpus luteum from the follicle wall after the egg has been released. The corpus luteum produces the hormone progesterone in addition to estrogen. If pregnancy does not occur, the corpus luteum has a natural life of about 12 days and will degenerate on about Day 26.

The endometrium in the uterus is very sensitive to the hormonal changes just described and goes through its changes in response to the ovarian hormones. During the first half of the cycle, as the follicle develops and estrogen is secreted, the endometrium grows and proliferates (proliferative phase). Following ovulation and under the influence of the progesterone produced by the corpus luteum, the endometrium prepares itself for the implantation of the egg (luteal phase). As the corpus luteum degenerates and the levels of estrogen and progesterone decline, the endometrium is broken down and sheds itself as the menstrual period. With the use of an endometrial biopsy we can follow these hormonal changes and the endometrial response very precisely. Alterations in this response can be a cause of infertility.

The mucus-secreting cells in the cervix are also responsive to the ovarian hormones, something that is most apparent just before ovulation— when the levels of estrogen are at their peak and the cervical mucus becomes very abundant, clear, and stretchy. (Many women describe midcycle mucus as having the consistency of egg white.) This type of mucus is favorable for the transport of sperm. Changes in the mucus are fairly easy to detect, and these observations are the key ingredient to many of the natural family-planning methods that allow avoidance of intercourse while midcycle mucus is present. As you have probably guessed, failure of the mucus to respond properly to the hormonal changes can also result in infertility.

THE BIRDS AND THE BEES

If intercourse has taken place around the time of ovulation and adequate numbers of sperm are delivered to the cervix, pregnancy may occur. The semen forms a gel following ejaculation that then liquefies in twenty to thirty minutes. Some of the sperm move into the cervical mucus within minutes. Uterine contractions propel the sperm up through the uterus, and sperm can be found in the tube in as little as four minutes. (This extremely rapid movement explains why douching is not an effective contraceptive method.)

The numbers of sperm are dramatically reduced as they ascend the genital tract. Most are lost by simply leaking out of the vagina. However, in the upper genital tract, many get eaten up by scavenger cells all along the reproductive tract (phagocytosis). Also, some are lost through the fallopian tube into the pelvic cavity. So the next time someone tells you that all you need is one sperm you will know what an understatement that is!

As the sperm are making their ascent the egg, surrounded by its cumulus cells, adheres to the surface of the ovary until the fimbria from the fallopian tube sweeps over the ovary and picks it up. The eggs are quite sticky and adhere to tissue pretty well. Delicate hairlike microscopic structures lining the tube (cilia) move the egg into the tube. Fertilization usually takes place in the outer portion of the tube (the ampulla). The sperm wedge themselves between surrounding cells and then a sperm will penetrate the zona pellucida. The zona then becomes impervious to penetration of a second sperm. Within fourteen to twenty hours fertilization is evidenced by the development of two structures consisting of the genetic material from the sperm and egg (pronuclei), and by about twenty-six hours the embryo will start dividing. The embryo will continue to divide in the tube until it is a compact cluster of cells (morula). Then the embryo moves fairly rapidly down the tube, arriving in the uterus three to four days following ovulation. It remains in the uterus, where it continues to divide and finally begins to implant in the endometrium about six days after ovulation. Certain cells of the embryo begin to secrete what we commonly refer to as pregnancy hormone (human chorionic gonadotropin, or HCG). The presence of HCG is sensed by the corpus luteum, which continues to produce progesterone. This prevents the endometrium from breaking down and the menstrual period from occurring. The corpus luteum will continue to function until the pregnancy can produce enough estrogen and progesterone to support itself.

MONITORING YOURSELF

Since much of what we have discussed relates to normal body functions, we want to make you aware of the signs to understand how your own reproductive system is working. All of these observations are safe, fairly simple to do, and (except for one) free of cost. In fact, some of the simpler ones are utilized by the natural family-planning methods to try to prevent conception. You can put them to use in helping you get pregnant by making your timing of intercourse optimal.

Monthly cycle

You can calculate your most fertile time based on the history of your previous cycles, especially if your menstrual periods are regular. Ovulation usually occurs about two weeks before the next expected menstrual period. This is because the luteal phase of the cycle usually lasts twelve to fourteen days. So if, for example, you have the often-quoted twenty-eight-day cycle, your ovulation probably occurs on Day 15 of the cycle. If your cycle is usually thirty-five days, ovulation will most likely occur on Day 22. If there is a variation of your cycle of never less than twenty-eight or more than thirty-five, you need to take that variation into account and you will probably ovulate between Day 15 and Day 22. It's easy to calculate, but you do need to know the variation of your cycle length. Remember, no woman is absolutely regular. Even some women who thought they were regular were actually irregular when cycles were closely observed.

Temperature chart

If you've had even the most preliminary infertility workup and treatment, you are probably familiar with the basal body temperature (BBT) chart. The concept is really quite simple. It was observed that one of the effects of progesterone on the woman's body is a slight temperature elevation of about a half a degree. A woman's temperature has the least variation day-to-day upon awaking, before any physical activity (basal temperature). Therefore the slight shift caused by progesterone is most noticeable at that time.

If you take your temperature first thing in the morning, before you get out of bed or go to the bathroom, and chart it for one complete menstrual cycle, you should see that *following* ovulation the temperature rises and stays up until just before the next menstrual period. You don't even need a special thermometer. A good-quality thermometer that you are able to read to one-tenth of a degree will do. If you have difficulty reading a thermometer, then one of the new electronic digital thermometers is for you.

You should not use the temperature chart to time intercourse. The temperature shift from the production of progesterone has a variable relationship to release of the egg and often occurs some time following ovulation, at which time it may be too late! You can sometimes see a slight dip in the temperature before ovulation, but this is not consistent and reliable.

We feel that the BBT is a valuable way for you to understand your cycle and can be used for scheduling and interpreting infertility tests. However, it is not very good for predicting ovulation. Some physicians do not advise its use at all because they feel that it adds to the anxiety and stress already present in the couple experiencing an infertility problem. Some use it on a limited basis (for example, for only three cycles) and then, once it has served its purpose, discontinue it. You can judge its value to you for yourself.

Cervical mucus

Like those women learning natural family-planning methods, you can learn to identify the cyclic changes in the cervical mucus. At the time of ovulation, the cervical mucus becomes abundant, clear, and elastic, with the consistency of egg white. Again, you can use this observation along with the regularity of your cycle and the results of previous months' temperature chart to determine your most fertile time of the month. You can check the mucus by observation or, if not enough is visible, you can check it by putting a finger into the vagina and sweeping it across in front of the cervix to obtain some mucus.

Monitoring the LH surge

Now we are getting more scientific. Over the past few years manufacturers have come out with home test kits for various medical conditions. One of the first and most prominent has been the home pregnancy test kit. There are now a number of these on the market; they give the consumer the opportunity of doing her own pregnancy test and obtaining the result privately.

The home testing trend now includes tests for detection of the LH surge. A variety of tests on the market utilize the detection of the LH surge in the urine, but we find Ovustick (now called Ovukit) to be the most reliable. Ovustick and Ovukit give a very clear-cut result, which is a blue color on a test pad on a stick. You match this result to a standard blue color resulting from a known concentration of LH comparable to that which would occur during the surge. The results are accurate, although it takes over an hour to perform. Many people like Ovuquick, which takes only four minutes. However, some women do not get as clear-cut a result with Ovuquick. Ovuquick, which employs a daily test strip with the standard and test on the same strip, seems to be more sensitive to increases in fluid intake. So, if the results are not clear, a more definitive endpoint may be reached if fluids are restricted during the period of time the test is being used.

We usually recommend that the test be done in the afternoon or evening, starting a few days before anticipated ovulation. We recommend doing the test later in the day because the surge most commonly starts in the early hours of the morning and then takes some time to reach levels detectable in the urine. If it is done in the morning, you could miss the surge that day and pick it up the next day, one day late. Remember, we are not detecting the beginning of the surge but detecting evidence that the surge started during the preceding twenty-four to thirty-six hours. Since ovulation usually occurs some thirty-six to forty-four hours after the beginning of the surge and we may be detecting it up to thirty-six hours after the surge has started, we recommend that couples have intercourse that evening or the following morning. If insemination is planned, we time it for the following morning.

PREPARING FOR PREGNANCY

There are some steps you should take before attempting pregnancy.

1. *Make sure you want to have a baby.* This may sound foolish, but many couples approach the attempt to get pregnant without giving a great deal of thought to the effects on their life of having a child. They say "Let's get pregnant" instead of "Let's have a baby." Creating a baby and being pregnant sound glamorous. It may be glamorous, but you should really want to have a baby. Don't get us wrong—we think having a baby is great. But is it great for you? You may think this never happens, but we see new mothers who say:

"If I knew what this would do to my life..."

"I don't know who is going to watch the baby so I can go back to work..."

"I didn't know how much it was going to cost to have a baby..."

"My husband didn't really want a baby and it's driving us apart..."

Make sure your relationship is strong. It's generally a serious mistake to have a baby to try to patch up a shaky marriage. You just compound your problems and it's certainly not the ideal way to bring a new life into the world.

2. *Learn all you can about your genetic history.* If there is any significant history of genetic problems in the family, you may want to investigate it before attempting to get pregnant. This could include a relative with Down's syndrome or other mental retardation, muscular dystrophy, cystic fibrosis, hemophilia, or other inherited diseases. You

may belong to a population group that carries an increased risk of diseases specific to that group, such as Tay-Sachs disease in Ashkenazic Jews or certain types of anemia in blacks or in people whose ancestors came from Mediterranean countries. This applies to *both* wife and husband. Your own doctor can help you with advice in this area or he or she will refer you to a place where you can get more information.

For example, we know of a Jewish couple, one of whom is a physician, who did not come in for care until about twelve weeks of pregnancy. They had never been tested for Tay-Sachs. They were sent to the local Tay-Sachs testing program and *both* turned out positive. By this time, she was seventeen weeks pregnant.

Since Tay-Sachs is a uniformly fatal disease with progressive neurological deterioration and death by age three, they were sent for genetic counseling. They were told that their offspring would have a 25 percent chance of having the disease and a 50 percent chance of being a carrier. Fortunately, it can be detected in the amniotic fluid and an amniocentesis (withdrawing amniotic fluid with a needle) was scheduled immediately. We were all relieved when the amniotic fluid revealed that the baby was not affected. But this is something that ideally should have been known and planned for before the pregnancy. In this case, if they had waited any longer and if the result showed an affected baby, they would have had no choice but to continue the pregnancy and subject the baby to the certain fate of Tay-Sachs.

3. *Clean up your act!* Both of you should get into the best physical shape possible. Stop all medically unnecessary drugs, especially recreational drugs, including marijuana. These can have an effect on fertility as well as on the baby. Avoid smoking and excessive amounts of alcohol or caffeine. Caffeine and smoking are both implicated in infertility. One study comparing smokers and nonsmokers going through in vitro fertilization found that the smokers had lower fertilization rates, lower estrogen levels, required greater amounts of fertility drugs, and had a lower pregnancy rate. Another study showed that a cup of brewed coffee daily was assoicated with a 50 percent reduction in the chance of conceiving each month. Effects on outcome with infertility treatments have not been studied. Other sources of caffeine are tea, colas, and chocolate.

Check at work for any environmental hazards to conception or pregnancy. If you are overweight, it is a good idea to lose the weight before you get pregnant and do it in a manner consistent with good nutrition. Then continue on a nutritionally sound weight-maintenance program. If your weight is normal or you are underweight, make sure that you are eating a well balanced diet. If strenuous exercise has made your periods irregular, you might want to modify your routine while trying to conceive. Finally, if your level of stress is a problem, you can try to avoid stress or use some stress-reduction techniques. Again, your doctor can be of help with this type of planning.

The effect of physical stress is well demonstrated by one of our patients, Barbara, twenty-eight, who had no difficulty conceiving her first child. Then after about a year of trying to conceive again, she came in quite concerned. A competitive rower, she had been training extensively for both individual and group events. In fact, she proudly appeared at one of her appointments with the gold medal she had recently won. All tests were normal except for one which revealed that she was not developing an adequate endometrium for implantation. She is currently winding down her training in order to see if she can spontaneously correct the problem.

4. *Consider taking vitamins daily.* In preparation for pregnancy, some authorities are recommending the use of vitamins containing the daily requirement for pregnant women. These are easily obtained over the counter at any pharmacy and are fairly inexpensive. There are many different brands, but all contain about the same formula. Do they help? It's not clear. A study from Boston, reported in *The Journal of the American Medical Association* in January 1990, suggested a much lower incidence of neural tube defects in women who took vitamins containing folic acid before conception. In any event, they can't hurt if taken as directed.

5. *Consider existing medical problems.* If there is any question of a medical problem, it is a good idea to have this evaluated and treated before getting pregnant. This is especially true if diabetes is present or suspected. Fertility will be greatest and the chance of fetal abnormalities will be minimized by starting the pregnancy with normal blood sugars. So we recommend that all diabetics be checked and get an okay from their doctor before even attempting to get pregnant. You should be sure that other medical conditions are under control and that medications to control them are appropriate for pregnancy, since some medications could increase the chance of fetal abnormalities.

MAXIMIZING YOUR CHANCES

As we will explain in greater detail later, a couple with normal fertility who have intercourse at or about the time of ovulation stands about a 20 percent to 25 percent chance that a pregnancy will result. In order to reach this level of maximum efficiency of the human reproductive system, be sure that:

- Intercourse occurs as close to the time of ovulation as possible.
- The man's sperm is at optimal levels.
- The environment is suitable.

Intercourse can be timed to occur on the day of ovulation as determined by the calendar, examination of previous BBTs, cervical mucus, or (for the more scientifically minded) the urinary LH home test. Precise timing may be more scientific, but it does tend to add stress to the process and after a while can even take the fun out of it. An alternative would be to be sure to have intercourse at least every other day. Given the life of the sperm and the egg, this would tend to have sperm present during the "life" of the egg no matter when ovulation occurs.

So why not have intercourse four times a day? That's fine, but that will tend to deplete the numbers of sperm produced by the man. Remember, we are talking about maximizing your chances of producing a baby. On the other hand, it is not a good idea to limit sex to "save it up" for one time, because that may reduce the motility (movement) of the sperm. Motility tends to decrease with longer periods between ejaculations. The best compromise appears to be a two-day interval to maximize your chances of conception.

By environment we do not mean candlelight, music, and wine. We are talking about position and the avoidance of practices that might be harmful to sperm. The man-above-woman-below position is best for most couples, with the woman staying on her back for about twenty minutes following ejaculation. The use of artificial lubricants and douching after intercourse should be avoided.

INFERTILITY

So far, almost all we have discussed pertains to normal reproduction and the couple who has no problem conceiving. So how do you know if you have an infertility problem? Infertility is defined as the inability to conceive a baby after one year of fairly regular unprotected intercourse. That's *not* the same as trying to have a baby for a year. For example, we have seen couples come in with a history of unprotected intercourse for several years, but they didn't think they had an infertility problem. We don't know where the notion that you have to be "trying" came from. If the factors controlling your fertility are normal and you are having unprotected intercourse, you will get pregnant whether you are "trying" or not.

In some couples, we reduce the period of time of unprotected intercourse to six months before considering them as possibly having an infertility problem. These might be couples who are in their late thirties or forties and who, for that reason, are anxious to conceive quickly. Also included would be those couples in whom we can identify a potential problem. But for most couples the rule of one year of unprotected intercourse applies.

After a review of the basics of male reproduction in Chapter 3, we will discuss the causes of infertility in Chapter 4. But don't skip Chapter 3. There are basics there you need to know, and—like eating your vegetables—it's good for you!

three
The Male Partner

Just as we stressed in Chapter 2 regarding the female, it is vital to understand the normal reproductive process in the male in order to be able to appreciate the complexities of the technology we describe later in the book.

OH, NO! NOT MORE ANATOMY!

The male partner is either the sole or a contributing cause of infertility in up to 40 percent of infertile couples, but his role in the fertility process has generally been understated until recently. Actually, the parameters to establish normal male fertility were not even developed until the 1950s, when normal semen was defined by Dr. J. MacLeod in 1000 fertile men and in 800 men in infertile marriages. However, with the advent of assisted reproductive technology, there has been renewed interest in the male's role in the fertility process. Much has been learned about male reproduction based on the procedures developed to enhance fertilization in the laboratory, and this knowledge is now being applied to conventional fertility testing and treatments as well as to advanced reproductive technologies.

ANATOMY

As in the female, we will be concentrating on the anatomy in two areas of the body—the base of the brain and the pelvis.

At the base of the brain is the pituitary gland, the master gland of the body, which controls many other glands just as it does in the female. However, in the male we are not concerned with a cyclic function like the menstrual cycle of the woman controlled by the hypothalamus but with the continuous production of the pituitary hormones.

In the pelvic and groin areas we find the male reproductive organs (Figure 3) consisting of:

- THE TESTICLES—the male's gonads, located in the scrotum. They consist of a compartment that produces sperm and cells (Leydig cells) that produce male hormone (testosterone).
- THE EPIDIDYMIS—a tubular network located at the top of each testicle. It leads sperm away from the testicle and consists of a single long, narrow coiled tube about 12 to 18 feet long attached to each testicle. The epididymis is about 1/300 of an inch in diameter.
- THE VAS DEFERENS—the next part of the tubal system. It is connected to the epididymis on each side and travels from the scrotum into the groin and ultimately empties with fluid from other reproductive organs into the urinating channel (urethra).
- THE SEMINAL VESICLES—add fluid to the semen, which aids ejaculation.
- THE URETHRA—a tube that is the urinating channel leading from the bladder to the outside, through the penis. The vas deferens and seminal vesicles on each side empty through the ejaculatory duct into the urethra in the region of the prostate gland.
- OTHER ORGANS—the prostate gland, Cowper's glands, and seminal vesicles all contribute fluid to make up the semen. In fact, the sperm cells make up only a small fraction of the total ejaculate.

PHYSIOLOGY

As in the female, the hypothalamus stimulates the pituitary gland to produce hormones that, in the male, instruct the testicle to produce sperm as well as male hormones, primarily testosterone. The pituitary hormones leave the gland and enter the blood circulation to reach the testicle. Although the pituitary hormones stimulate both sperm development and testosterone production in the testicle, these are independ-

Male reproductive organs

1	bladder	7	spermatic duct
2	seminal vesicle	8	epididymis
3	raphe	9	glans
4	prostate	10	foreskin
5	erectile tissue	11	testis
6	urethra	12	anus

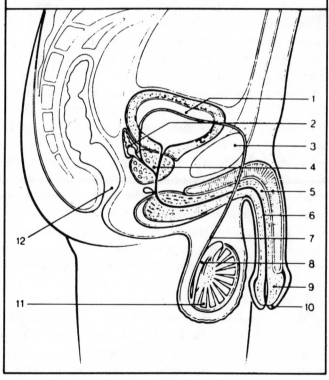

Figure 3

ent functions, and it is common for abnormalities to exist in sperm-producing areas of the testicles with normal production of male hormones. The two pituitary hormones are the same as in the female but are not cyclic. Follicle-stimulating hormone (FSH) primarily stimulates the production of sperm, while LH is responsible for stimulating Leydig cells to produce testosterone. This differs from the female, where they must be produced in the proper sequence to cause ovulation.

Sperm begin as very simple cells and go through prolonged phases of development to reach maturity. They are manufactured in tubelike structures called seminiferous tubules. Initially, immature sperm cells are round, but as they mature they elongate and assume the typical tadpole appearance of a mature sperm. The sperm consists of:

- A head, containing all the genetic material
- A middle part to provide energy needed for movement
- A tail that moves to propel it forward

The sperm travel from the testicle through the epididymis into the vas deferens. The vas deferens takes them from the scrotum into the groin and ultimately empties them with the secretions from the other reproductive organs into the urethra. Actually, there are two complete systems, one on each side, which both empty into a single urethra. The urethra, which usually carries urine from the bladder to the outside, has a muscle at the outlet of the bladder that closes, normally preventing the ejaculatory fluid (semen) from going back into the bladder at the time of ejaculation (retrograde ejaculation). With contraction of these muscles, the fluid in the urethra has only one way to exit—through the penis. A tiny amount of fluid from small glands at the base of the penis (Cowper's glands) is added to the semen and appears at the tip of the penis just prior to ejaculation.

When the sperm leave the testicle, they are fully formed but have no motility (movement). As they travel the entire length of the epididymis, they acquire motility and complete their maturation. It takes about seventy-two days for the sperm to begin its development and progress through complete maturation. Any abnormality in this complex system can result in subfertility or infertility. Since it takes almost three months for sperm to develop fully and be transported, it stands to reason that any treatment which improves sperm production can take up to three months to be reflected in the ejaculate.

Near the seminiferous tubules are the Leydig cells, which produce testosterone. This hormone is responsible for the development of all the masculine characteristics: deep voice, male hair pattern, heavy musculature. Since different cells produce sperm and hormones and different pituitary hormones stimulate the two different functions, it is common for a man to be fully masculine yet have a problem producing sperm.

WHAT MAKES A GOOD SPERM?

There are a number of parameters used to determine the quality of a sperm sample. Actually, some of these criteria may not directly relate to sperm function and, despite the fact that a specimen may appear perfectly normal, there may be other factors that may prevent the sperm from fertilizing an egg. Some common parameters used in the complete semen analysis are:

- Sperm density—the numbers of sperm in a milliliter (cubic centimeter) of ejaculate (over 20 million per milliliter is considered normal).
- Morphology—categorizing sperm by their shape. Every man has some abnormally shaped sperm in the ejaculate. In fact, it is considered normal for up to 50 percent of the sperm to be shaped abnormally. There is no evidence that these abnormal forms increase the chance of birth defects. They are simply less able to fertilize an egg.
- Motility—represents the percentage of sperm which are moving (at least 40 percent is normal). The degree of motility is assessed and varies between 1 + (shaking in place) and 4 + (progressive forward motion). Newer computer-assisted semen analysis actually measures their velocities and even the quality of motion.
- Viscosity—an evaluation of the thickness of the semen after a period of time following ejaculation when the semen should become more fluid (liquefy). If the semen fails to liquefy, the sperm may not migrate well into the cervical mucus.
- Volume—the total amount of the ejaculate (varies from 1 to 5 milliliters). If the volume is too low, the sperm may not reach the cervix.

MAXIMIZING YOUR CHANCES

In Chapter 2 we discussed many of the ways a woman could monitor her menstrual cycles and advised ways to maximize the couple's chances of conceiving. There is no such advice directly applicable to men with the exception of general advice such as avoiding X-rays or excessive heat to the scrotum, medications and drugs (especially recreational drugs); avoiding smoking, excess alcohol, excessive stress, and toxic agents such as pesticides and industrial chemicals. The combination of caffeine intake (four cups of coffee a day) with smoking (more than twenty cigarettes a day) has recently been shown to cause significant decreases in sperm motility and increases in numbers of dead sperm. Excessive and chronic alcohol use also has a harmful influence on sperm development.

Excessive heat to the testicles can be prevented by not using heated spa-type baths or tight-fitting clothing like briefs. However, changing underwear from briefs to boxer shorts has never been *proved* to improve fertility, and if a man is uncomfortable with looser-fitting shorts most experts in male fertility would not recommend a change.

INFERTILITY

Just because a man is sent for a reproductive evaluation does not mean that he has an abnormality. He is simply a partner in a couple with reproductive delay. The evaluation of the semen by various other techniques will be described later and will further define the liklihood of his being a contributor to the reproductive problem.

It is normal for a man's semen to be quite variable even on a day-to-day basis. For this reason, when a man is evaluated for reduced semen quality, at least three specimens should be obtained before drawing any conclusions. Also, it is necessary to wait at least three months between collecting groups of samples in order to see a real change resulting from treatment because of the time required for maturation and transportation of sperm.

Now that you have the basic knowledge needed to understand the information in the rest of the book, you can move on to Chapter 4, where we consider what types of problems can cause a delay or inability of a couple to conceive.

four

When It
Doesn't Work

"It's as American as Motherhood,
Apple Pie, The Flag, and Baseball."

Y ou grow up, go to school, get married, and start a family.
Not necessarily. At least not for the 10 to 15 percent of
American couples for whom motherhood or, more correctly, parenthood, does not come so easily. These are the couples plagued by
infertility. For many reasons, the least of which may be that the couple
does not meet the expectations of well-meaning friends and relatives,
trying to solve an infertility problem can be a humiliating, demeaning,
and totally frustrating experience. It can even lead to the end of a
relationship.

A common perception among infertile couples is that everyone else
they know is getting pregnant. But this is probably a misconception. It
seems a cruel irony that in 1988, just as the birthrate for the United
States climbed to its highest point since 1964, the Office of Technology
Assessment (OTA) was reporting that an estimated billion dollars was
spent the preceding year on the treatment of infertility. So, not *everyone*
else is really getting pregnant even if it may look that way.

Provisional data released by the National Center for Health Statistics
show that an estimated 3.9 million babies were born in the United
States in 1988. That is 2 percent higher than the number reported in
1987, which puts us in the midst of a minor baby boom. Yet the same
year the OTA was reporting that 2.4 million couples were plagued by

infertility and that the number of visits to physicians for infertility had *doubled*, from one to two million, in the past several years. Are we, therefore, in the midst of a baby boom and an infertility epidemic at the same time?

We can actually count how many babies are born each year. If we add those 3.9 million babies to the Centers for Disease Control (CDC) estimate of 1.3 million abortions being performed every year, we can even get a fairly decent count of how many women are getting pregnant. However, we cannot determine with any accuracy if there is an infertility epidemic because we can only roughly estimate how many couples are currently infertile in the United States. We do know there is an increasing demand for infertility services. But is it because more couples are actually infertile, or has more awareness of the availability of new reproductive technologies brought more infertile couples in for treatment?

Many experts feel that, instead of an infertility "epidemic," there's merely greater demand for services based on more effective treatment, a recognition of infertility as an acceptable problem, and the increasing willingness of insurance companies to consider infertility a medical problem and pay for its treatment. We may actually be witnessing both an increase in the incidence of infertility and an increased demand for services.

SOCIAL FACTORS THAT INCREASE INFERTILITY

It makes sense to postulate a true increase in infertility when you examine the social forces that tend to result in more infertility.

Delayed childbearing—the chronologic age factor

This is perhaps the most frequently quoted reason for our "infertility epidemic." Anyone who has been practicing obstetrics during the past twenty years cannot help noticing a dramatic change. The norm twenty or more years ago was for women to finish their secondary education, get married, and have a baby in their late teens or early twenties. Now that situation is less commonplace and we are seeing many women finishing advanced education, developing a career, and becoming financially stable before thinking of having a baby. By the time they accomplish all this they are often in their mid-thirties or early forties. Suddenly, it seems, they realize that it is time to start a family before time passes them by.

A widely accepted notion is that age alone is an important factor in a woman's ability to become pregnant. This is based on a 1982 French study which led to the perception that *all* women in their early to mid-thirties are at risk for infertility if they delay childbearing. The study reported that fertility rates (the ability to become pregnant) in women who were never previously pregnant declined from 74 percent before age thirty to 62 percent between ages thirty-one and thirty-five and down to 54 percent by age thirty-six. According to these data, by ages thirty-one to thirty-five fully one-third of women would not get pregnant. And, by age thirty-six, almost half will be barren. That's pretty scary if you're over age thirty-five and trying to conceive. But there's a problem with these results. They were obtained *only* in women who were never previously pregnant and then were applied to *all* women. This invalidates the study, since a group of women who have never gotten pregnant may be infertile for reasons other than age.

Another problem with this French study was that it was conducted only in women undergoing twelve cycles of artificial insemination by a donor. That eliminated any fertility effects due to frequency of intercourse or husband's fertility. Even though the donors were all assumed to be fertile, it is felt that twelve cycles of artificial insemination would not yield as many pregnancies as one year of intercourse.

An English study of women who have previously had babies and thus have proven fertility found that age alone does not increase the risk of infertility significantly until age thirty-eight. This is in general agreement with the 1982 National Family Growth Survey, which showed increases in infertility rising from 10.6 percent at twenty to twenty-four, 13.6 percent at thirty to thirty-four, and only dramatically rising to 24.4 percent at ages thirty-five to thirty-nine and then to 27.2 percent at forty to forty-four. Now, that's in women who had previously been pregnant. For those women who are trying to decide whether they can space their children, it is reassuring that the effects of age alone are not so dramatic as to deny them that luxury.

What is the sum total of the effects of age on fertility? The studies quoted above looked only at the effect of age in women *without* a known fertility or other problem when they first attempted pregnancy and did not indicate the chance of the older woman who has a fertility

problem becoming pregnant. In studies of treatments in older women
who have failed to conceive, the effects of age have been fairly
dramatic, often reducing success rates by more than 50 percent.

Delayed childbearing—other factors

It would stand to reason that delaying childbearing would allow
other conditions such as gynecologic disease and medical conditions
which might afflict an individual to occur as time passes. By far the
most important would be gynecologic disease, primarily pelvic endometriosis, and to a lesser extent tubal disease and adhesions as the
result of pelvic infection from sexually transmitted diseases. We'll
discuss these conditions in greater detail later in this chapter. But first,
let's take a brief look at them as they relate to delay in childbearing.

The delay itself

A delay in childbearing itself would appear to lead to infertility since
previous childbearing confers protection against infertility. Over the
twenty years studied, the National Family Growth Survey found a
decrease in the infertility rate from 19 to 13 percent in women who
became infertile after having one child. In contrast, they found an
increase from 16 to 22 percent among those women who had never had
a child. The rate in women with two or more children remained
constant at a low 10 percent. We do not know why there was this
apparent decrease in infertility in couples who already had a least one
child. It may have been because these couples are monogamous and
therefore less likely to contract a sexually transmitted disease. It is
possible that childbearing protects against gynecologic disease, or
perhaps there may be some as-yet-undiscovered factor.

Sexually transmitted diseases

We have certainly witnessed a change in sexual mores over the last
two decades, with a resultant epidemic of sexually transmitted diseases.
It was estimated at the beginning of the 1980s that there were more
than 212,000 annual hospitalizations for pelvic inflammatory disease.
Studies have shown that 11 percent to 12 percent of women will be
left infertile after one episode of tubal infection. The figure rises to 23
percent after two episodes and goes above 50 percent after the third.
The number of hospitalizations does not even take into account the
patients who are treated in doctor's offices or those left untreated. In
addition, some infections, particularly chlamydia, may silently damage

the tubes. In fact, about half the women we see with tubal occlusion have no history of any infection in the past.

IUD use

In the late 1960s and early 1970s the IUD—intrauterine device— enjoyed increasing popularity. The newer devices were made from plastic instead of metal, as were the earliest devices designed in the 1930s. They were relatively inexpensive and came into wide use. By the time it was discovered that they predisposed the wearer to pelvic infection, many women had suffered irreparable damage to their tubes, especially from the Dalkon Shield IUD.

Endometriosis

Endometriosis is a disease that is most likely caused by chronic retrograde flow of menstrual blood back through the tubes. In some predisposed women, fragments of endometrium may implant and grow around the tubes and ovaries. These implants are stimulated by the normal monthly fluctuation of hormones to undergo cyclic changes. Over time the disease creates enough inflammation and scarring to interfere with fertility. Early occurrence of a pregnancy and birth interrupts this process, probably by decreasing retrograde menstrual flow as the result of widening the cervical opening. In addition, the pregnancy treats any areas of the disease already present. Endometriosis is called "the career woman's disease"; women who have a child early in their reproductive years are seldom afflicted.

Uterine fibroids

These benign muscle tumors of the uterus increase markedly in frequency and size with age. Depending upon their location, they can reduce the chance of conception, increase fetal loss, or require surgery—which can cause scarring. A fibroid growing under the lining of the uterus can make the environment less receptive for implantation or, as it may grow rapidly during the pregnancy, can put pressure on the expanding pregnancy and can cause miscarriage or premature birth.

Gynecologic surgery, ectopic pregnancy, therapeutic abortion

As time passes, there is more chance for the development of an ovarian cyst or other problem that could require surgery. Incisions in the ovary tend to cause adhesions around the tube and ovary that can impair fertility. If an unwanted pregnancy occurs, not only could the rare complications of an abortion impair future fertility, but a pregnancy could lodge in the fallopian tube, resulting in loss or damage to that side. If ovulation is only occurring half the time next to a healthy tube, obviously the chance of a normal pregnancy occurring in any one month is decreased markedly.

Premature ovarian failure

The ovaries can start to fail many years before the average age of menopause (fifty-one). If this occurs, the chance of stimulating residual eggs in the woman's ovaries is small. In smokers, the average age of menopause is four years earlier, and since the ovaries can show signs of impaired function years before the menses cease we can safely say that "smoking and delayed childbearing don't mix!"

How should these complex factors affect your decision of when to start a family? We advise that you not delay unless there is a strong reason, particularly if a fertility problem has already been identified. We have seen too many couples who have waited until "everything is perfect" only to find that the one thing most important to them forever eludes their grasp.

In any event, what we are seeing clinically is more women in their thirties and forties who want a child but are unable to get pregnant. But if there are so many couples dealing with infertility, why do you feel alone?

YOU ARE NOT ALONE!

While there may be another 2,399,999 couples struggling with infertility, that is little solace for the couple facing this problem. First, it is little relief to know that others are suffering with you. Second, couples with infertility do not usually share their problem with others, so we might think of these couples as a "silent minority." The highly visible majority are the people who have gotten pregnant. An example of their high visibility is something we all have experienced, standing in a supermarket line in back of a woman with a newborn baby. As you may or may not be admiring her new offspring, her eyes meet yours and you feel compelled to say "My, what a cute baby!" They seem to be everywhere!

She will probably use your statement as a cue to tell you the gory details of her labor and delivery. But then are you going to say "Did you know that I really want to have a baby, but I can't? My tubes are blocked!" Probably not. When it doesn't work and you have not met the expectations of friends, family, and society in general, it is something you, and others like you, do not generally go public with.

Not too many years ago, at public health forums in local hospitals subjects such as heart disease, cataracts, breast cancer, and even sexual problems would draw them out in droves. But when the subject was infertility, only a handful of people showed up. They would listen intently, not asking many individual questions. When asked why attendance was not better, many said that their friends who were also having difficulty conceiving would not come because they did not want to acknowledge publicly that they had this problem. The more recent and healthier trend is for more couples to "come out of the closet" with their infertility as evidenced by the development and growth of support groups like RESOLVE, Inc. Sharing any medical problem with family, friends, and others with similar problems is a more productive way of dealing with the problem because it allows you to get some important emotional support.

WHY IS THERE SO MUCH INFERTILITY?

Human reproduction in its unassisted form is remarkably inefficient. Substantial embryonic loss is a routine part of the life cycle among humans and in fact among all mammals. Most eggs are never fertilized and, if fertilization occurs, as many as one fourth to one third of human conceptions end in miscarriage, for reasons that are poorly understood.

Testimony of **Gary B. Ellis**, Ph.D. Senior analyst, Office of Technology Assessment, at Congressional sub-committee hearing on Consumer Protection Issues Involving In Vitro Fertilization Clinics, March 9, 1989

Reproduction is basically a very inefficient system. After all, it takes millions of eggs in the woman and billions of sperm in the man to create perhaps a handful of offspring during their lifetimes. Consider for a minute what would happen if General Motors did business this way. If it took millions of engines and billions of bodies to create a few automobiles, it would not be long before GM would be out of business.

What actually exists in the human reproductive system is a dichotomy. You have portions of the system with a fantastic amount of reserve and margin for error. At the same time, portions of the system rely on the successful completion of minute details, any one of which can prevent the system from working. After all, there is not one ovary, but two. In these two ovaries there are not only the 500 or so eggs a woman will need for her reproductive life, but there are hundreds of thousands at puberty. On the other hand, the portion of the system that controls implantation of the embryo into an adequately prepared endometrium relies on:

- A precise sequence of hormones to prepare the endometrium
- Receptors in the cells of the endometrium to accept the proper hormones
- Cellular functions controlled by complex codes to make the cell respond in the proper fashion

Thus we are slaves to a system that contains gross excesses and at the same time precise mechanisms which can be foiled by the slightest alteration in function.

WHAT CAUSES INFERTILITY?

There is a great deal of variation in the incidence of the major causes of infertility among centers in different parts of the country and, in fact, even in areas of the same city serving different populations. Although these figures may vary from those in your area, it will be useful, just as an example, to look at the primary factors responsible for infertility in one large study reported in 1980, reviewing over 600 cases. Figures in other studies may vary considerably. But this study found the primary causes to be:

	Percent
Endometriosis	25
Male factor	18
Lack of ovulation	15
Tubal problem	12
Luteal phase problem	7
Cervix or mucus problem	5
Uterus problem	2
Other problems and unexplained	16

Lack of ovulation

The first requirement for a successful conception is the meeting of two germ cells. A woman's lack of ovulation (anovulation) deprives the system of the female germ cell and foils attempts at conception at the most basic level. Treatment directed to the specific cause of the anovulation can promptly lead to pregnancy.

We can look at anovulation as occurring at three basic levels in the female reproductive system. It can occur as the result of failure of either:

- The ovaries
- The reproductive centers in the brain and pituitary
- Malfunction in the interactions among parts of the reproductive system resulting in a disruption in the orderly sequence of hormonal changes which controls the maturation and release of the egg

Ovarian failure

Failure of the ovaries prior to the usual age for menopause is termed premature ovarian failure. This is relatively easy to diagnose by measuring the level of gonadotropins. In premature ovarian failure, these are very high, perhaps two- or threefold of normal. This results from the hypothalamus and pituitary gland overreacting to a lack of feedback signals from the ovaries. When the hypothalamus senses that the ovaries are not responding, it reacts by stimulating more and more gonadotropin to try to make the ovaries respond. Thus we find the gonadotropins markedly elevated. Occasionally the ovary can be made to respond by first suppressing the level of gonadotropins, which may restore a degree of consistency of response of the follicles. This would then be followed by administration of gonadotropins to try to evoke a normal ovarian response. If this is not effective, donation of eggs from another woman may be considered.

Brain and pituitary problems

In patients with failure of the reproductive centers in the brain or pituitary, we find that despite adequate and properly timed signals, the hypothalamic–pituitary axis is unable to respond. This would occur, for example, in the patient who has a pituitary tumor interfering with pituitary function. Such a tumor (or simply an overactive pituitary) can secrete excess amounts of the hormone prolactin, which then suppresses the hypothalamus. Prolactin also stimulates the breast to secrete milk, a symptom called galactorrhea. Prolactin levels can be minimally elevated with either no galactorrhea or only some minor menstrual irregularity. It is possible that small increased amounts of prolactin can prevent conception even without any measurable effect on the ovulatory process.

An example: Sally, thirty-seven, and John, thirty-eight, went through the usual workup for infertility, including a laparoscopy. Then they switched to a local infertility clinic with a good reputation, and went into higher-level tests without finding any problem whatsoever. Despite the fact that she was ovulating normally, Sally was tried on a course of fertility drugs combined with artificial insemination. As a last resort before going into one of the high-tech procedures, her physician recommended a thorough evaluation of her hormones even though her ovulatory function appeared normal. Sure enough, her prolactin was mildly elevated, about 50 percent above normal levels. Since a proportion of women with elevated prolactin have a small pituitary tumor called a microadenoma, her doctor ordered a special scan to examine the pituitary gland. They found a small microadenoma of her pituitary gland. The drug bromocriptine (Parlodel) was administered to shrink the tumor and suppress the elevated levels of prolactin. Two months after starting treatment, her prolactin was normal and she became pregnant on her own without any other treatment.

The other common central defect is malfunction of the hypothalamus, the area in the base of the brain that sends out the signals that control the pituitary gland. Reduced function of the hypothalamus, resulting in reduced secretion of gonadotropin-releasing hormone, may be due to stress, anxiety, excessive exercise, crash dieting, and anorexia nervosa. Gonadotropin levels may be normal or reduced and menstruation can be infrequent or absent.

Failure of normal interactions

The most common problem of signal interaction is polycystic ovarian disease (PCO), sometimes called Stein-Leventhal syndrome. In PCO, the adrenal gland and the ovaries produce increased male hormones. The fat tissue in the body converts these to female hormones at an increased rate. This constant increase of estrogen disturbs the functions of the pituitary, which secretes increased levels of LH. This increased LH causes the ovary, in turn, to secrete increased amounts of male hormones. Follicles develop only partially. This results in numerous small cystic follicles within the ovary, giving the syndrome its name: polycystic ovarian disease. PCO can be suspected by a lifelong history of infrequent or absent periods, with or without increased hair growth or excess body weight.

A group of symptoms that may signal an ovulatory problem includes:

- Lack of a period (amenorrhea)
- Irregular periods, especially less than a twenty-one- or more than a thirty-five-day cycle
- Abnormal hair growth
- Lack of menstrual and premenstrual symptoms
- Severe acne
- Breast secretions

Needless to say, it is very important to relate any of these symptoms to your physician when he or she takes your history. Given modern medicine, except for premature ovarian failure most women with anovulation can be treated successfully with conventional measures.

Male factor

The other gamete necessary for conception is the sperm. In general, problems in the male have been thought to contribute to infertility in up to 40 percent of infertile couples. In the large study mentioned above, male factor accounted for 18 percent. Despite the significant percentage of couples in which the male factor is important, until recently the male had been relatively ignored in the workup. With the development of a subgroup of physicians interested in the study and treatment of male reproduction (andrology) in conjunction with the use of new assisted reproductive technologies, new developments in the conventional workup and treatment of the male have occurred.

When the male factor is evaluated, the most important principle is that it be done with an eye toward making a specific diagnosis in order to be able to implement specific therapy. Unfortunately, there are circumstances when a specific diagnosis is not achievable. When this situation occurs it should be discussed openly and frankly and the choices for nonspecific therapy evaluated.

The conditions most frequently associated with male infertility were studied in a male infertility clinic among 425 men. These conditions were found to be associated with this group of infertile patients to the following extent:

	Percent
Varicocele (enlarged veins in the scrotum)	37.4
Low sperm count—no apparent reason	25.4
Failure of the testicles	9.4
Blockage of the ducts leading from the testicles	6.1
Undescended testicles	6.1
Inadequate semen volume	4.7
Agglutination (clumping together of sperm)	3.1
Sexual problem	2.8
Semen too viscous (thick)	1.9
Could not ejaculate	1.2

Each of the remaining causes occurred in less than 1 percent of the men. We cannot be sure that some of these conditions are the precise cause of the infertility in a particular couple. For example, there is some controversy over the importance of a varicocele in causing infertility in some couples.

The urologist may categorize the male partner in the couple by the results of the semen analysis. He or she will find men falling into one of three categories:

- Semen analysis is normal
- Semen analysis is abnormal
- Not sure whether there is a significant abnormality

Normal semen analysis

The man with normal semen analyses is unlikely to be the sole cause of the couple's infertility. Additional tests may be necessary, because the normal semen analysis eliminates only the possibility that a drastic problem exists. More subtle problems regarding the sperm's ability to travel through cervical mucus and penetrate an egg may still be present in the face of an apparently normal semen analysis. Therefore the specialist may not end the evaluation here, but rather go on to some of the newer tests of sperm function, most of which are unrelated to any specific cause we can yet identify.

Abnormal semen analysis

Azoospermia If there are *no* sperm present whatsoever, the physician must consider hormone tests to differentiate among an obstruction of the duct system, testicular failure, and pituitary malfunction.

Other abnormalities The man with one single or many parameters abnormal in the semen analysis might have one of the conditions mentioned above such as a varicocele, which is an engorgement of the veins surrounding the testicles in the scrotum. These dilated veins in the scrotum can cause impaired sperm function by mechanisms not yet completely understood. Less common causes of abnormalities in the semen may be external environmental factors. One of the most common single abnormalities we see is asthenospermia, a reduction in the motility of sperm below 40 percent to 50 percent of the sperm present. If this, for example, is combined with some clumping of the sperm, the physician might suspect the presence of sperm antibodies.

Not sure It is normal for normal men to have significant variability in the results of their semen analysis from day to day. Most urologists will not hang their hat on one result and will want two to three analyses to compare. Even after looking at the results of multiple specimens, they may not be sure if there is an abnormality and will want to test further.

Tubal infertility

Now that we have considered the production of the two germ cells, we have to get them together. The fallopian tube is where the two gametes normally come together. Diseases that cause tubal blockage can prevent conception for mechanical reasons. These tubal problems are important because of the large numbers of patients affected, numbers that seem to be increasing. In the 1980 study cited above, tubal factors accounted for 12 percent of infertile couples. With the sexually transmitted disease (STD) epidemic of the last two decades, we are seeing a rise in this problem to where it is now thought to be a factor in up to 20 percent of couples experiencing infertility.

The "classic" STD that causes tubal damage is gonorrhea. The organism spreads through the cervix and endometrium to the fallopian tube, where it causes salpingitis (infection in the tube), often referred to as PID (pelvic inflammatory disease). If untreated or inadequately treated, PID can frequently progress to form an abscess. These processes often can damage tubal function, result in partial or complete obstruction, and lead to either infertility or tubal pregnancy. The final stage of the pathologic process is the development of a hydrosalpinx. That's where the tube becomes a distended, fluid-filled sac that is often not amenable to successful surgical repair because even if the tube can be opened, it may not function properly.

More recently, with the advent of better culture techniques, we have learned that an organism called chlamydia is very frequently associated with the occurrence of milder degrees of salpingitis. One of the most dangerous features of chlamydia is the fact that this organism causes an insidious type of infection that is frequently unrecognized and does its damage silently. Many women with tubal damage from chlamydia cannot recall a distinct episode of tubal infection in their history. In addition to tubal obstruction, these infections can cause adhesions to form in the pelvis around the tubes and ovaries. In some cases the tubes may appear open on X-ray dye tests, but scar tissue surrounding the tubes and ovaries may prevent the egg from reaching the tube.

One of the more recent important causes of pelvic adhesions was the resurgence of the use of IUDs in the late 1960s and early 1970s. Of particular note is the story of the Dalkon Shield IUD, a device released by the A. H. Robins company with the claim that its unusual shape would prevent one of the more common problems with other IUDs, expulsion from the uterus.

To prevent it from being pushed out of the uterus, it was shaped something like a crab, with several small "claws" on its side to help retain its position in the uterus. These claws prevented its expulsion but also made it more difficult to remove. Most IUDs were attached to a string that hung down through the cervix into the vagina to facilitate removal. These were usually made of a monofilament nylon similar to fishing line. Because a stronger string was needed due to its shape, the Dalkon Shield had a string made of multifilament nylon rather than the usual monofilament nylon. It is now thought that it was the multifilament nylon string that caused the infections seen with this device. The string acted as a wick, bringing bacteria from the vagina into the upper genital tract.

An example of how previously "hopeless" tubal damage can be overcome by assisted reproductive technology is well illustrated in the story of Cheryl and Jeff Scruggs. Cheryl, twenty-seven, and Jeff, twenty-eight, came in with a history of nine months of infertility. Their history was unremarkable, but Cheryl was anxious to the point that she was convinced that something had to be wrong. Although we usually advise a young couple to try for a year before starting any tests, Cheryl didn't want to wait until that long. So a workup was started including a tubal dye-X-ray test. In view of her negative history it was surprising to find that her tubes were not only blocked but were also distended with fluid. When this was confirmed by laparoscopy, it was determined that her tubes were damaged beyond repair. Because of the poor chance of success afforded by tubal surgery, Cheryl and Jeff elected immediately to try in vitro fertilization, which would bypass the need for tubal function. Their first cycle was not completed because the development of scheduling problems, but in their second try they had twin girls. (More about the details of these procedures appears in Chapter 7 and there is more about Cheryl and Jeff in Chapter 10, where we follow them through their IVF cycle.)

Endometriosis

Endometriosis was the most common cause of infertility in the study cited above, possibly because it is one of the most common gynecologic disorders seen in women in the reproductive age group. Even before the advent of sophisticated tests and procedures to determine the causes of infertility, this condition was clinically associated with impaired fertility.

Endometriosis is the presence of endometrium, the normal lining tissue in the uterine cavity, growing anywhere outside the uterus. It is normal-appearing tissue that belongs in the cavity of the uterus and is simply somewhere else. Most likely, that somewhere else is the ovary or the lining of the pelvic cavity, but it could (and does) occur anywhere else in the body. That may include the bowel, appendix, or even the elbow! But it is the presence of endometriosis on the organs of the pelvis that results in infertility.

It can either be a silent disease or cause severe symptoms. The most common symptoms are worsening menstrual cramps or pain, particularly starting before menstruation, and pain with intercourse. In some cases, there are no symptoms whatsoever except otherwise unexplained infertility. One of the most interesting aspects of this condition is that the amount of endometriosis present does not correlate with the degree of symptoms. For example, it is common to see women with no symptoms turn out to have a pelvis filled with endometriosis. It is just as likely to find a person with very severe menstrual cramps and pain having only a tiny bit of endometriosis present and to have those symptoms relieved when the condition is treated.

Typically, small amounts of endometriosis look like burn marks on the affected tissue, almost as if someone had burned the tissue with the head of a match. Larger degrees of the disease will look like brown, raised areas, or when it affects the ovary a "chocolate cyst" (endometrioma) will result. This will be a variably sized fluid-filled sac replacing all or part of the ovary that oozes a brown, chocolatelike material when the cyst is opened. All of these manifestations occur because the endometrial tissue bleeds, just as it does in its normal location in the uterus, and the old blood in the tissues turns a dark red-brown.

Endometriosis tends to run in families, as evidenced by the fact that in one study siblings of patients with endometriosis had a 7-percent incidence of the disease. It is thought to develop primarily in women who have delayed childbearing.

Various theories have been proposed to explain how the endometrial tissue gets where it's not supposed to be; the most likely is the back-up of menstrual fluid and tissue. Another possible explanation is that some cells in the body have the potential to turn (differentiate) into endometrium. What we do know is that when the endometriae tissue gets where it's not supposed to be it mimics the same hormonal pattern of the endometrium in the uterus. These endometrial implants grow as the cycle progresses and then "menstruate" at the end of the cycle. As the implants break down and bleed, you can see how they could cause pain. Since they damage the ovary, they can impair ovarian function and cause menstrual disorders. Also, in cases of severe endometriosis, the presence of large endometriomas and scarring can literally block the pick-up of the eggs by the fallopian tube. But even small amounts of endometriosis can inhibit fertility. Recent research has proposed a number of possibilities of how the disease interferes with fertility. One possible mechanism is a greater number of cells that pick up debris (scavenger cells) in the pelvic cavity. In patients with endometriosis, they are also more active than usual in scavenging sperm. Since the number of sperm gathering around the egg is a balance between the numbers succeeding in reaching the tube and the number being removed, this increased scavenging of sperm reduces the chance of the sperm and egg meeting. Other possible mechanisms include inflammatory substances that injure the sperm or embryos or that can interfere with the development and release of the egg, or an allergic-type response to the endometrial tissue that may interfere with the normal uterine lining.

Luteal phase defect (LPD)

The second half of the menstrual cycle following ovulation, the luteal phase, is critical to the success of the process. The egg can meet the sperm, fertilization can take place, and the resulting embryo can be transported down the fallopian tube and into the uterus. But, if the endometrium is not prepared to receive the embryo for implantation, the whole process will literally be aborted.

Following ovulation, progesterone must be secreted in adequate amounts and the endometrium must be capable of responding. If the hormones are not correct, the luteal phase could be shorter than necessary, so that the menstrual period begins shortly after the embryo is ready to implant. Another possibility is that the amount of progesterone may simply be inadequate to produce an orderly maturation of the endometrium coordinated with the arrival of the embryo to help it implant. In turn, the embryo must implant adequately to secrete pregnancy hormone (human chorionic gonadotropin or HCG), which will "rescue" the corpus luteum from its normal demise so that it continues to produce estrogen and progesterone, which in turn support the pregnancy.

Although the number of patients with this problem is not large, it is impressive that treatment often works and is generally neither risky nor expensive. These patients are the ones in whom we look for some other subtle hormone problem such as an elevated prolactin level.

Cervix or mucus problem

Another less common but treatable cause of infertility is a problem with the functioning of the cervix. It may involve blockage of the cervical canal and/or deficiencies in the production of the all-important cervical mucus necessary to transport the sperm across the cervix. In addition, the mucus has a function in preparing the sperm for fertilization (capacitation). Infections of the cervix, congenital abnormalities, or the presence of sperm antibodies are all factors that can reduce the ability of the mucus to transport the sperm. Another less frequent cause of the cervical factor is previous surgery on the cervix, such as a cone biopsy done to evaluate an abnormal Pap smear. This surgery can result in scarring that can reduce the production of cervical mucus and/or cause a stricture (stenosis) of the canal. Finally, women who were exposed to DES in utero, if they develop infertility, are more likely to have poor cervical mucus.

To fully evaluate the cervical factor, it is helpful to evaluate the interaction between the mucus and the sperm. The couple is therefore asked to have intercourse the night before or on the morning of the test. (If having to perform on schedule makes you unable to complete this part, that's a normal reaction; simply tell your doctor. He can still evaluate the mucus.) If you do have intercourse, male fertility factors can influence the results. For example, impotence, inability to ejaculate normally, and certain anatomical abnormalities of the penis such as urethral opening on the shaft instead of at the tip (hypospadius) may give a bad result. Other male factors previously discussed can also result in a poor outcome on the mucus test. Most often, however, deficiencies in the amount and viscosity of cervical mucus, as well as the presence of infection or antibodies in the mucus, account for the problems related to the cervix.

One of the most common causes of an abnormal test is simply poor timing. Timing this test is not easy, since women are generally less regular than they realize. In order to assure that the test is timed to coincide with peak mucus quality, we now recommend the use of simple and accurate self-tests for urinary LH (Ovukit, Ovustick).

Uterine factor

Although the uterine factor is relatively rare as a cause of infertility (2 percent), again we have a factor that in some cases is treatable. For example, fibroids can be treated by surgery. These are exceedingly common benign tumors of the uterine muscle. In fact, it is estimated that by age thirty-five about one-third of women will have clinically detectable fibroids. For the vast majority of women, these fibroids have no effect on their ability to become pregnant or carry a pregnancy to term. But the fibroids that are large or classified as submucous can cause problems. These are the tumors which push into and distort the cavity. They can interfere with sperm transport and can interfere with the blood supply of the endometrium and prevent implantation, as well as put pressure on the expanding pregnancy. It is thought that they may also act as a foreign body in the endometrium which can prevent pregnancy in ways we do not fully understand. In this regard they may act in the same manner as an IUD intended to prevent pregnancy.

But we must be careful not to accept fibroids as the only cause of infertility until all other causes have been eliminated. In fact, distortions of the uterine cavity have been associated more with early pregnancy loss and late miscarriage than with infertility.

The second treatable uterine condition that is occurring more frequently is the development of adhesions in the endometrial cavity. These are usually the result of previous surgery, specifically a D&C (dilation and curettage) related to the termination of a pregnancy. Adhesions can occur if termination of the pregnancy was induced by therapeutic abortion, or they can arise spontaneously after a D&C following a natural miscarriage. It can also happen after a D&C unrelated to pregnancy. Suspicion of this condition would arise if a menstrual period did not occur after such an operation, or if the menstrual periods became scanty following a D&C. At times, enough adhesions can exist to prevent pregnancy but allow normal menstruation. These adhesions can be treated surgically by means of a telescopic device (hysteroscope) placed into the uterus through the cervix.

Certain malformations of the uterus, such as the presence of a septum dividing the endometrium, could be included in this category and can be removed through the hysteroscope. These malformations are also more likely to result in frequent pregnancy loss than in infertility.

Infections are the third treatable uterine condition that can lead to infertility. But these are not the usual infections we see that lead to tubal scarring. These infections include less common organisms such as ureaplasma and even tuberculosis. These can cause a long-standing (chronic) infection in the endometrium. Ureaplasma infections are treatable with common antibiotics. Tuberculosis as a cause of infertility, rare in the United States except in immigrant populations, is more common in developing countries. Medical treatment of the infection will not resolve the problem and the tubal scarring caused by the infection is not correctable by surgery, leaving IVF as the only option.

The one uterine factor that, unfortunately, is not treatable is prenatal exposure to diethylstilbestrol (DES). DES is a synthetic estrogenic hormone but is different from estrogen because it has a different chemical structure. It was a popular practice among obstetricians twenty to thirty years ago to give large doses of DES to women who were threatening to miscarry or who had a history of previous miscarriage. It was thought that the extra estrogen would help the woman retain the pregnancy.

However, it was becoming clear by the early 1970s that the female offspring of women who took DES in pregnancy were experiencing certain specific problems. The first problem to be recognized was a dramatic increase in a rare type of vaginal cancer in a group of young women. As the story unfolded, it was noted that these offspring also had specific changes in their vagina, cervix, uterus, and fallopian tubes. The changes in the uterus and tubes are the ones most pertinent to fertility and pregnancy loss. These uteri often have a narrowed, irregular, T-shaped cavity that does not accommodate a pregnancy well and leads to miscarriage or premature labor. The tubes may also be malformed. Except for documented obstruction of the tubes, it is not known if such DES changes per se are a direct cause of infertility, except that tubal pregnancy is more common. As mentioned, there is no specific treatment for these DES changes, so patients with this problem need to have all the other aspects of the fertility process studied and treated. They can frequently be successful, but they should be made aware of the problems they may experience in carrying a pregnancy. Because of this, we tend to advise longer courses of those treatments that do not tend to increase the chance of multiple pregnancy or are easily repeated if the pregnancy is not carried to viability.

Unexplained infertility

As our knowledge of the fertility process improves the number of couples in this category decreases. Currently about 5 percent of couples should fall into this category, given our present level of knowledge. These are the couples who have been completely worked up medically and in whom all tests are normal. Perhaps, as we continue to increase our knowledge, unexplained infertility will finally disappear. For example, many women whose infertility has been classified as unexplained have an increased population of scavenger cells in the abdomen near the tubes and ovaries, presumably resulting in fewer sperm available to fertilize the egg. Currently the only way we can clinically recognize this factor in a woman with unexplained infertility is if she conceives readily after a tubal X-ray using an oil-based dye that inhibits those scavenger cells.

Psychological and emotional factors

The significance of an emotional factor is controversial. We have all heard of the couple who achieved a pregnancy after adopting a baby or, like the Meldrums, after going away on a long vacation. This is the common advice given infertility patients: "Just relax! When the pressure is off, it'll work." Often it is given by well-meaning friends and relatives. Sometimes it even may be given by health care professionals before a full evaluation has been performed. And, at times, it is given following a complete evaluation that has shown no apparent cause of the problem. But does the desire to become pregnant along with the seeming inability to achieve this goal result in sufficient emotional and psychological upheaval to prevent pregnancy?

The answer is a definite maybe. We all know that having difficulty in conceiving a baby and going through the process of evaluation and treatment are tremendous stresses for each individual and for the couple together. They have to confront feelings of failure, inadequacy, guilt, and loss of self-esteem that may lead to marital and family conflict. Some of the evaluations and treatment may even make matters worse. The couple's sex life may be strained by the demands of "sex by the calendar." The man, who may not have been too pleased about having to go through it all just to have a baby, may become fed up with the necessity of coming to the doctor's office, being handed a plastic cup, and being told to perform. He may even tire of wearing boxer shorts to cool his testicles. And so, by the time the couple is many months or even years into the process, infertility becomes an obsession that may truly impair their lives and their relationship.

But can that stress affect and prolong the infertility? There is only anecdotal evidence that it can. For some couples, abandonment of the attempt to become pregnant quickly resulted in a successful pregnancy. Most reproductive experts know of such cases. But there is no scientifically valid data to support this occurrence. On the contrary, the positive effect of adoption was refuted in a fourteen-year study at

Stanford. They followed 895 infertile couples and found that the ultimate pregnancy rate was not statistically different between couples who eventually adopted and those who didn't.

A TYPICAL PATIENT

A profile of a typical patient struggling to get pregnant with multiple factors (endometriosis, luteal phase defect, cervical factor, and perhaps psychological factors) is exemplified by Penny. She and Roger were married for seven years before she first tried to become pregnant at age thirty-six. Tests by a doctor in another city showed evidence of endometriosis with fairly large cysts on the ovaries (endometriomas). An operation removed her left tube and ovary, which were beyond repair, and all but a sliver of her right ovary. She then moved into our area and wanted to continue her quest. This was before assisted reproductive techniques were readily available. So her treatment was geared toward monitoring her cycles for ovulation, treating her luteal phase defect with fertility drugs, promoting better cervical mucus with small doses of estrogen, and checking by means of laparoscopy to be sure her endometriosis had not returned. But by age forty-one she felt that she had had enough of temperature charts, fertility drugs, and sex-by-the-calendar and she decided to stop trying. Her son, Brett, was born just short of her forty-second birthday.

Which factor was actually preventing her from becoming pregnant? Age? Endometriosis? Cervical factor? Luteal phase defect? Psychological pressures? Did her giving up have anything to do with her conceiving? We will never know.

The other story you will hear is that after adopting a baby a couple with years of infertility treatment conceived. It sounds like this strategy may work. Actually, what you do not hear about are the vast majority of couples who do *not* conceive after adoption. Remember that Stanford study that found no difference in the conception rate between couples who adopted and those who did not. Therefore our advice is not to abandon testing and treatment with the hope that adoption or other change in life style will work. Pursue both at the same time and you will have your maximum chance of success!

Now that you understand the major causes for a couple not being able to achieve a pregnancy within a reasonable period of time, we will move on to the process for finding the problem in an individual couple. "So, first we have to do some tests!"

five

First, We Have To Do Some Tests

PATIENT: *We have been trying to have a baby for a year and nothing has happened.*

DOCTOR: *First, we have to do some tests!*

What a scary statement. No matter what the medical problem, the prospect of having to undergo tests that could be painful, expensive, and even dangerous strikes fear into the hearts of even the most brave among us. The fear surrounding the tests themselves does not even take into account the dread of what those tests might reveal.

"Maybe I can never have a baby."

"Perhaps the test will show that it's my fault and my husband/wife will resent me ... or even leave me, and I will be all alone."

"If they find that I have no sperm, maybe I'm not really a man."

All too often the need for testing in this very sensitive area can bring out underlying marital and psychological problems. For example, Stephanie, thirty-four, came into the office with the concern that she and David, thirty-six, have been trying to have a baby on and off for about two years. She appeared quite anxious about this problem. Her medical and reproductive history did not reveal an obvious cause for their difficulty. The physical examination was equally unrevealing. Only when the process got to the point of outlining which tests would be suggested for the initial part of the workup did we appear to hit upon the source of her anxiety.

When we mentioned the need of a semen specimen from David, she tearfully recounted that David did not really want a child. He agreed to have a child if she wanted to, but now that they were having trouble, he would not cooperate in any way with the infertility workup. He told her that it was probably her problem, anyway. Further discussion led to the discovery of significant marital problems. Shortly after they were referred to a psychologist for marital counseling, they separated. According to the psychologist, their difficulty surrounding the decision to have a family was merely an indication of deeper troubles in the marriage.

Today their friends believe that their breakup was due to the stress caused by the infertility, when in fact the marriage was on shaky ground before the infertility problem surfaced. Happily for her, Stephanie remarried and had no difficulty conceiving. David remarried, to a woman who shared his feelings about not having a family.

We feel that one can learn a lot about a couple by watching their interaction as various tests and procedures are suggested. Excuses and delays by either party or the couple together may indicate a less than enthusiastic commitment to starting or expanding a family.

BEFORE THE TESTS

Actually, tests are not the first step the doctor takes. The first step should be a thorough medical history of the couple as well as an in-depth review of their reproductive history. If you go to see a doctor who, after hearing that you have difficulty getting pregnant, immediately suggests a laparoscopy to see if your tubes are open, this is not the doctor for you. And if he or she recommends one of the assisted reproductive technology (ART) procedures at this point, head for the door!

Most doctors have their own order for scheduling the tests. The common thread through all their regimens will be that the safer, simpler, less invasive, and less expensive tests should be done first. This reserves the more invasive, expensive, and risky tests for later. And later may never come. You may get pregnant before the later arrives. The safest, simplest, and least expensive part of the evaluation will be the history—which is where all doctors should start.

PREPARING FOR THE FIRST VISIT

We will give you some of the topics about which you will be asked so that you can search out the answers you may not know off the top of your head. Also, if this is not your first visit to a doctor for this problem, bring with you any documentation you have regarding previous tests and procedures. Actual X-ray films are better than descriptive reports. If an operation has been done, bring a copy of the operative report. Actual laboratory values for hormone tests are infinitely better than "My thyroid was normal, I think." Seeing semen analysis results will help the doctor determine if it was done properly and thoroughly. If, for example, you had a laparoscopy with video, ask your previous doctor to loan you the video or copy it for you. A picture is worth... Well, you get the point!

TOPICS AND QUESTIONS

Either the doctor or nurse-practitioner-coordinator may ask the questions. In addition to the usual medical and surgical history from both of you, they will want to know about routine medications you take and any allergies you may have. Now, medications will include drugs, and drugs include anything you put into any part of your body that cannot be classified as food. It is *very* important to reveal any recreational drug use, since some of these compounds can have an effect on your reproductive system. The doctor may not ask about these drugs in so many words, but realize that it may be important, so offer the information even if not specifically asked. This also goes for significant medication you may have taken in the past. This is a good question to ask your mother before the visit, since you might not have been told what you were given as a child. These could include chemotherapy for cancer or DES given to your mother while you were in utero, either of which could have significant implications for your fertility.

For example, Lorraine, twenty-four, and Steve, thirty-two, were concerned about their ability to have a child because Steve received chemotherapy for an early cancer in a testicle several years before. He was warned by the oncologist that although adequate treatment of the cancer would probably lead to a long life for Steve, it would be at the cost of his ability to have children. When tests confirmed that he was, indeed, sterile, they decided to try artificial insemination with a donor's sperm. They carefully selected a donor who matched Steve's physical and educational characteristics from a list supplied by the regional sperm bank. The first insemination resulted in a pregnancy and the birth of a healthy boy about six weeks before term. They were so delighted with the result that they had the sperm bank reserve a quantity of the same donor's sperm for the time when they would want to expand their family. Lorraine recently delivered their second child, another boy.

Occupational history may be very important, too; some occupations involve contact with environmental factors that can affect reproduction. An office worker is less likely to run into this type of problem than is an engineer at a toxic waste dump. But if you do come into contact with noxious chemicals in your job, find out what they are before the appointment and present the physician with a list of them so he can check them out for you.

Social habits may provide some clues to the cause of a couple's fertility problem. For example, unusual amounts of exercise can have a profound effect on the female reproductive system to the point that marathon level runners frequently may not even menstruate. Other runners and aerobic exercisers of lesser magnitude may have less dramatic, but potent, effects on their fertility. In men, practices that can lead to heating of the testicles are thought by some to diminish fertility. Smoking is a very important social habit: not only can a significant delay in fertility in women be related to smoking, but the overall fertility rate is also reduced by 30 percent. A recent study reported from the University of North Carolina showed that drinking four or more cups of coffee and smoking more than a pack of cigarettes a day had a deleterious effect on sperm motility and increased the percentage of dead sperm.

Previous reproductive history for both individuals is most important. This includes not only previous pregnancies by the couple together or with others but also prior contraceptive history. For example, the use of an IUD may be a clue to unrecognized tubal problems. The history can sometimes get a little sticky since there may be something which either of the parties may not want revealed to the other—a child with another partner or, more likely, an abortion. Whereas we usually encourage candor with one's partner, you can divulge anything in confidence to the doctor, even if you do not feel able to reveal it to your spouse. If you are worried that your spouse may see copies of the chart, ask the doctor not to write it in the record. He or she is obligated to keep anything you wish confidential.

For the female, there will be specific questions relating to menstrual cycle. These will include age of onset, interval between periods, length of periods, associated menstrual symptoms such as cramps and pre-menstrual symptoms. Other questions relating to the pelvic organs may include whether she has the common physical signs of ovulation or pain with intercourse.

Sexual history of the couple together will be explored. This may include inquiries regarding frequency and position of intercourse, the use of artificial lubricants, and douching after intercourse. Many physicians have had the experience of solving an infertility problem at this point merely by teaching the couple proper timing or eliminating the use of a sperm-toxic lubricant or douche.

THE PHYSICAL EXAMINATION

Once the history has been obtained, the next safest and most cost-effective part of the workup is the physical examination. At this time, it is the woman who gets examined. In fact, most of the time it is the female partner who comes in for the initial visits. We encourage the male partner to come in for the first visit, help provide the history, and be there to support his wife through these tests and procedures.

The physical exam is not unlike the complete physical you may get every year from your family doctor, internist, or gynecologist. There will be more emphasis on the pelvic examination, of course. The physician will be looking for signs of infection in the cervix that might give a clue to infection in the tubes, evidence of endometriosis, or any of the various problems discussed in Chapter 4.

THE TESTS

At this time, we would expect that the doctor would sit down with you in the consultation room and explain the series of tests. We like to think of these tests as being done in phases. Again, the tests with the least risk and cost will usually come first; if necessary, the more expensive and invasive tests will be done later. Since all infertility specialists do not recommend the tests in exactly the same order, you can expect some variation. Just keep in mind that safer, simpler, less expensive should come first.

We will rate them against each other as to risk, pain, and cost from NONE to LOW, MEDIUM, and HIGH. It is not possible for us to give specific and accurate estimates of costs for all these tests and procedures because there is tremendous regional variation; it would be best for you to determine average costs of key procedures when you make your initial search for a provider.

In general, in the patients without any significant history, our testing would be phased as follows:

> **PHASE 1**
> Basal body temperature chart
> Semen analysis
>
> **PHASE 2**
> Tubal dye test (hysterosalpingogram)
> Postcoital test
> Endometrial biopsy
> Serum progesterone
>
> **PHASE 3**
> Laparoscopy
> Other tests

PHASE 1

Basal body temperature chart (BBT)

Most of the fertility tests will be timed to your menstrual cycle; in order to do this we have to monitor your cycle. One of the simplest ways of doing this is by utilizing the basal body temperature chart (BBT) (Figure 4). The basal temperature, the lowest temperature of the day, is fairly constant. Once you get up and engage in any activity, there will be a significant and variable increase in your body temperature. The BBT takes advantage of the principle that after ovulation the secretion of progesterone causes a half-to-one-degree rise in your temperature, most evident in your basal temperature. Thus the BBT can show if and when you are ovulating and the length of each phase of the cycle. All you need is a good-quality thermometer which you can read to a tenth of a degree (for example, 98.7). You can use a digital-readout thermometer if that is easier for you, but you do not need to invest in a special "basal thermometer."

You can make up a chart starting with the first day of your period as Day 1. You then take your temperature each morning, as soon as you wake up, *before* you get out of bed, when it reflects a true basal reading. Have the thermometer at the bedside, take your temperature immediately upon awaking, and record it on the chart in the column next to the appropriate date. If you can't wait to empty your bladder, keep the thermometer in a styrofoam cup in the bathroom and urinate into the cup. The temperature of the urine will be the same as your body temperature and you can read the thermometer anytime.

After you have done this for one or two months, the doctor can review the chart and probably tell if and when you ovulated, whether you had intercourse at the correct time of the cycle to maximize your chance of getting pregnant, and whether there was adequate time following ovulation for an embryo to implant in the endometrium before your period.

Some physicians do not use the BBT at all since they feel that the daily gathering and recording of this information may increase stress and that this information can be obtained in other ways. Others use it on a limited basis, for just a few months, then discontinue its use once ovulation has been established and the patient has learned about the timing of her menstrual cycle. (RISK—NONE; PAIN—NONE; COST—NONE)

Semen analysis

Just as we need to learn that the woman is producing eggs, it is equally important to find out if the man is producing adequate sperm

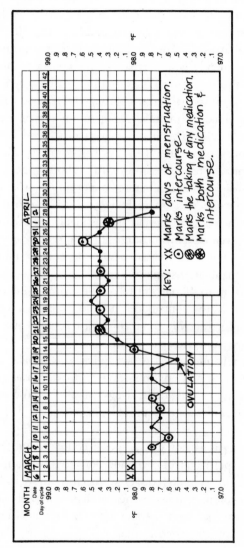

Figure 4

to achieve a pregnancy. To determine the man's status, a complete semen analysis will be obtained. If the doctor does not have his own reproductive laboratory, the male partner will usually be referred to a specific laboratory to have this done. At the lab or at home, he will masturbate a specimen into a special collection cup. It is best to have adequate sexual arousal before and during collection, otherwise a poor specimen could merely be an artifact of the collection procedure. One study showed that many male factors disappeared when the specimen was collected in a special sheath during intercourse. The laboratory should provide reading materials and an unhurried atmosphere. At home the wife may help with the collection. It is advisable to abstain from ejaculation for two to three days before the test in order to get his best specimen. This is because with a shorter interval the sperm density may be lower. But more importantly, will enable us to standardize the collection interval in order to compare results more accurately. With a longer period of abstinence the sperm may have lower motility. We usually recommend he give the specimen around the time of his wife's menstrual period since it is unlikely that she would get pregnant at that time.

We find that up to 40 percent of couples with an infertility problem have some male factor contributing to the couple's infertility. It does not make sense for the wife to go through tests that may involve some risk, discomfort, and expense if we don't at least find out if her partner's semen is adequate. In fact, physicians usually obtain several samples since health and environmental factors such as fatigue, smoking, stress, and use of caffeine or drugs can affect the results. Variation is *expected*, and only with repeated specimens is a full evaluation obtained.

A semen analysis is not just a sperm count (quantity) but also an assessment of sperm quality. In addition to the number of sperm present in a certain volume (count), we need to know the total amount of the semen (volume), how viscous or liquid it is (liquefaction), the number of sperm moving at various rates at different times (motility), and the shape of the sperm (morphology). Some laboratories also perform a mucus penetration test as part of the evaluation of the semen in which the distance the sperm can swim into a sample of a cow's mucus is measured. This measurement can generally be correlated with the ability of the sperm to penetrate human cervical mucus and might provide a clue to a condition in the man relating to sperm-mucus interaction. (RISK—NONE; PAIN—NONE; COST—LOW)

The results of the semen analysis will be placed into one of three categories:

1. Normal. This result most frequently represents reproductively normal men, but a small group of men whose semen appears reproductively normal have abnormalities of sperm function detectable only with more sophisticated testing.

2. No sperm found (azoospermia). This result should not only be confirmed with three specimens but should also be checked by two specimens that have been centrifuged, since azoospermia can be confused with a specimen with only a few sperm (marked oligospermia) if they have not been carefully evaluated.

3. Abnormal, but with sperm present. These men will have to be evaluated, as we discuss later in this chapter.

PHASE 2 (ABOUT ONE MONTH LATER)

Postcoital test (PCT)

We now move on to slightly more sophisticated tests. The postcoital test involves the examination of cervical mucus under the microscope for the presence of moving sperm after the couple has had intercourse just before or at the time of ovulation. The timing of this test is most crucial to its accurate determination of the quality of the sperm–mucus interaction.

Since proper timing is so vital, in addition to the BBT we often have the patient use one of the urine tests to determine the LH surge as the means for assuring precise scheduling of this test. Otherwise repeated visits may be necessary; often a poor test is simply due to poor timing. The LH surge will occur the day before ovulation, when the cervical mucus should be most favorable for sperm transit.

There are a number of test kits available both from doctor's offices and in the drug stores. Research has shown Ovustick (now called Ovukit) to be the most accurate. The most important instruction regarding this test is that the urine be tested in the afternoon or early evening. This is because the surge most often begins in the early morning; if you do the test too early you might not pick up the surge until the next day. A color change from white to a blue darker than the standard indicates that the surge took place that day and that ovulation should take place the next day.

The couple will generally have intercourse the morning following the detection of the surge and then the woman will come into the office for an examination of the cervical mucus for the presence of sperm. This is a very important test because it shows whether there is enough mucus, the quality of the mucus, and if her spouse's sperm can get into and survive in the cervical mucus.

Many couples ask if they should have intercourse any special way in order to have a better result on their PCT. The answer is no, because we want to be able to tell whether there are enough motile sperm in the cervical mucus based on their usual coital technique. (RISK— NONE; PAIN—NONE; COST—LOW)

Endometrial biopsy

The second test usually obtained in this phase is the endometrial biopsy. This test can tell if a woman is ovulating, the level of hormones in the second half of the cycle, and the response of the lining of the uterus to these hormones as it prepares to accept an embryo to implant. A normal result indicates that the whole system is functioning properly from the hormonal point of view.

The test is usually done eleven days after the surge is detected. (If the menstrual period occurs before the eleventh day, the cycle is too short and a problem exists.) The patient is positioned as for a pelvic examination. A thin plastic tube is placed into the uterus and suction is applied to draw in a small amount of endometrial tissue. The main concern is that if the patient is pregnant at the time, the pregnancy could theoretically be interrupted if the biopsy disturbed the implanting pregnancy tissue. Fortunately, this almost never occurs. In fact, the rate of miscarriages of pregnancies in cycles in which an endometrial biopsy was done is no greater than the average miscarriage rate.

The biopsy sometimes results in cramping, but we now use a smaller and more flexible instrument, which reduces the discomfort. Some physicians routinely use premedication or inject a local anesthetic beside the cervix. Prophylactic antibiotics may be used to prevent infection. Since there can be some variation in any woman's cycle, this test may have to be done more than once to insure consistency,

especially if the result is not perfectly normal. (RISK—LOW; PAIN—
LOW TO MODERATE; COST—LOW TO MODERATE)

Serum progesterone

Some doctors obtain a blood level of the hormone progesterone
instead of the biopsy. It is easier than the biopsy since it only requires
obtaining a sample of blood, but yields much less information.
(RISK—NONE; PAIN— NONE; COST—LOW)

Tubal dye test (hysterosalpingogram) (HSG)

We usually obtain a tubal dye test (hysterosalpingogram) just after a
menstrual period is over. You will generally be referred to a radiologist
since this test involves X-rays, although some gynecologists do their
own HSGs in conjunction with an X-ray department in a hospital.

This test involves a pelvic examination similar to a Pap smear. But
this time a small instrument is placed through the cervix into the lower
part of the uterus and some dye is injected. The radiologist will follow
the dye with a fluoroscope and take pictures as he or she sees the dye
go through and out the end of the tubes. This will allow visualization
of the contours of the endometrial cavity to determine if there might
be an abnormally shaped uterus, polyps, or fibroids. The radiologist can
see not only if the tubes are open and look healthy but also if the
pattern of the spill indicates there may be adhesions in the pelvis.
Another potential benefit is that if your tubes are open, the doctor can
inject a small amount of a special oil-based dye that, according to a
UCLA study, may help you get pregnant during the six months
following the test by inhibiting the ability of scavenger cells in the
pelvis to engulf sperm.

Cramping is fairly common with the injection of the dye, but you
can be premedicated with a mild tranquilizer and given a prophylactic
dose of a pain medication to help prevent or minimize the pain. If you
are particularly concerned, you can also simply take two ibuprofen
tablets (Nuprin, Advil, Medipren, Motrin) one hour before the procedure. Prior to having this test some physicians order a sedimentation
rate blood test to look for evidence of a previous pelvic infection,
indicating the possible need for antibiotic treatment before evaluating
the tubes. It is our routine to always use prophylactic doxycycline so
that even rare infections in women with normal tubes will usually be

prevented. (RISK—LOW; PAIN—MODERATE; COST— LOW TO MODERATE)

PHASE 3 (FOUR TO SIX MONTHS LATER)

Laparoscopy

This phase consists of a thorough look at the woman's reproductive organs by means of an operative procedure called laparoscopy. Before going on to this procedure, we usually wait four to six months after the HSG to allow for its therapeutic effect by reducing the activity of pelvic scavenger cells in patients with unexplained infertility and endometriosis.

The woman is usually admitted to an outpatient surgical center or the outpatient surgery department of a hospital. The procedure is usually done under general anesthesia but can also be performed with a spinal, epidural, or even local anesthetic. A small incision is made in the navel and a telescopic device is placed through this incision to look at all the internal reproductive organs. A small cut is made in the pubic hairline to insert another instrument to move the organs around so all aspects can be visualized. A dilute solution of dye will be flushed through the fallopian tubes by means of a small tube placed into the uterus through the cervix. This way the doctor can see not only if dye comes through the tubes but also that there is no scar tissue around the ovaries and tubes. With the anesthetic there is no pain felt during the operation, but there may be some minor discomfort afterward. Carbon dioxide gas is used to expand the abdomen to enable visualization of the organs. Although as much CO_2 as possible is removed, a small amount may remain and cause a bloated feeling and shoulder pain for a few days.

Although the HSG evaluates the inside of the tubes, there are other conditions that may be preventing pregnancy, such as adhesions or endometriosis, conditions which we have no other way of finding except by directly looking in the pelvis. The tubes can be open and yet adhesions around the ovary can block the egg from getting to the tube. Also, if adhesions or endometriosis are found at laparoscopy, there is a good chance that they can be corrected through laparoscopic surgery at the same time as the diagnostic laparoscopy. As in any operation, there are rare surgical risks such as bleeding or injury to bowel or bladder as the instruments are inserted and the organs manipulated. But the risk is small and the recovery period usually only a few days. It is recommended that the laparoscopy be performed before going on to even more sophisticated tests or treatments.

Some doctors now combine this laparoscopy with hysteroscopy. That is, at the same time they insert a telescope into the uterus through the cervix to make sure there are no congenital abnormalities, fibroids pushing on the cavity, or scarring. There is controversy over whether this adds any information to a normal HSG.

Laparoscopy is one of the most common operations performed by gynecologists. Many insurance plans will cover the procedure even if it is done to evaluate infertility. But be careful; some insurance policies specifically exclude procedures done to evaluate or treat infertility. If an insurance policy does exclude infertility but some other condition such as endometriosis or pelvic adhesions are discovered, the insurance may cover the procedure on that basis. Nowadays many plans require precertification, or even a second opinion, and may even pay better in a particular hospital or surgicenter. We recommend that patients contact their insurance company before having the operation to make sure they are eligible for the best benefits. (RISK— MODERATE; PAIN—MODERATE; COST—HIGH)

"WE FOUND A PROBLEM"

There are a number of areas in which problems may be found during the workup. The most common conditions encountered include:
- Problems with ovulation
- Problems with the semen
- Fallopian tube obstruction
- Pelvic adhesions
- Endometriosis

Ovulation defect

About 10 percent of patients demonstrate some defect in the ovulatory cycle. This could range from a history of lack of or infrequent menstrual periods, irregular cycles, evidence of lack of ovulation or short luteal phase on the temperature chart, or suggestion of a luteal phase defect on the endometrial biopsy.

For these patients the physician will probably initiate a series of blood tests to determine the source of the problem in order to specifically correct it. These may include:

- Serum FSH
- Serum LH
- Prolactin
- Testosterone
- DHEA-sulphate

Specific combinations of results from these tests can indicate the probable cause of the ovulatory problem and can help suggest therapy tailored to overcome the problem at its root. It is seldom necessary to do all of these tests. Depending on the clinical setting, usually one or two will suffice. (RISK—NONE; PAIN—NONE; COST—LOW TO MODERATE)

Semen problems (male factor)

Whether the semen analysis is normal or abnormal in any or several of its parameters, it needs to be repeated several times to determine if the results are consistent, realizing that it is normal for the semen analysis to show some variability. If the abnormality does show up repeatedly, referral to a urologist or an andrologist (a physician specializing in male reproductive problems) will be a likely next step.

The specialist in male infertility will begin, as in the female, by taking a history—including a sexual and reproductive as well as a general medical history. Of particular interest will be:

- REPRODUCTIVE
- Previous pregnancies fathered
- History of undescended testicles
- Operations performed on the testicles
- Genital trauma
- Mumps after puberty
- Hernia operations
- Bladder surgery
- Delayed puberty treated with hormones
- MEDICAL
- Diabetes mellitus

- Urinary tract infections
- Environmental exposures to chemicals, radiation, or heat, including high fevers within three months of semen collections
- Current and past drug use, including chemotherapeutic agents, recreational drugs, anabolic steroids, and all prescribed drugs
- SEXUAL
- Venereal disease
- Other infection
- Prostate gland infection
- Trauma to or infection of the scrotum
- Sexual dysfunction such as impotence
- Exposure to diethylstilbestrol (DES) as a fetus

In addition, special questions that help to assess any hormone abnormality focus on:

- Visual problems, particularly blind spots
- Change in frequency of shaving
- Abnormally sparse sexual hair
- Whether a normal sense of smell is present
- Change in physical strength

Again, as with the female partner, the next step will be the physical examination with special attention to signs of a hormone problem or genital abnormality. The examination will focus specifically on:

- Physical proportions
- Male hair distribution
- Presence of abnormal amounts of breast tissue
- Abnormalities of epididymis, vas deferens, or prostate
- Size and consistency of testicles
- Signs of enlarged veins in the scrotum (varicocele)

(RISK—NONE; PAIN—NONE; COST—LOW TO MODERATE)

The remainder of the tests to be done depend upon which parameters of the semen analysis are abnormal. Absence (azoospermia) or almost total lack of sperm (marked oligospermia) can result from obstruction of the ductal system in the testicle or a significant developmental or hormonal problem. If one or several parameters— count, motility, and/or morphology—are abnormal, a less serious hormone problem, environmental cause, or stress would be suspected.

Hormone tests similar to those done in the female partner would be indicated in the case of azoospermia. Since azoospermia may occur because of lack of pituitary stimulation, tests may include blood tests for levels of FSH, LH, testosterone, or occasionally prolactin. Again, as in the female partner, the combination of results will give the doctor a clue to the cause of the abnormality. For example, if a man has an elevated FSH and LH and a low level of testosterone his problem may be failure of the testicles. (RISK—NONE; PAIN—NONE; COST— LOW TO MODERATE)

With azoospermia a biopsy of the testicle may be recommended. The biopsy is an outpatient surgical procedure with minimal recuperation required. (RISK—LOW; PAIN—LOW; COST—LOW TO MODERATE) Unfortunately, if the biopsy confirms that no sperm are being produced, no treatment is possible and the couple will have to consider either donor insemination or adoption. This situation may arise because of absence of sperm-producing cells, trauma, mumps after puberty, or exposure to toxic agents. If adequate sperm are present on biopsy and hormone levels are normal, the problem is likely due to a congenital abnormality or acquired obstruction of the duct system and a scrotal exploration may be necessary to find the location. Although this is done on an outpatient basis, it is a longer procedure, depending upon what surgical procedures might be necessary to correct the obstruction, and more lengthy recuperation may be necessary. (RISK—MODERATE; PAIN—MODERATE; COST— MODERATE TO HIGH)

Obstruction can occur at any level beginning just within the testicle and progressing through the epididymis, vas deferens, and ejaculatory duct. Some men have a congenital absence of the duct system or it can develop as the result of injury, infection, or as the consequence of surgery. At times, the tubular system is present but functioning abnormally. This can occur with spinal cord or other neurological injuries or conditions that affect the ability of the bladder neck to close at the time of ejaculation. If the bladder neck fails to close, the ejaculate that enters the urethra flows back into the bladder (retrograde ejaculation) and leaves the bladder at the time of the next urination. This occurs most commonly in diabetes and following bladder-neck surgery.

In a man with a history of vasectomy reversal, infection, or testicular trauma, tests designed to detect antisperm antibodies in the blood or seminal fluid may be useful. Tests designed to detect infection with common organisms (such as chlamydia or ureaplasma) also might be employed. (RISK—NONE; PAIN—NONE; COST—LOW)

Finally, a sperm penetration assay (SPA) might be performed. This is more commonly known as the hamster test, because it records the percentage of hamster eggs penetrated by a man's sperm. The ability of sperm to penetrate the shell around the egg (zona pellucida) is usually specific to a particular species. In the hamster this shell can be removed by the use of enzymes, which allows the penetration of human sperm. In general, penetration below 10 percent is considered abnormal. However, the test results are not that specific, since pregnancies occur in couples with an abnormal hamster test (even those in which the SPA is zero) and some men who fertilize hamster eggs very well cannot achieve pregnancies. We therefore generally reserve this test until ART procedures are contemplated, since in vitro enhancement of fertilizing capacity may be possible. (RISK—NONE; PAIN—NONE; COST—MODERATE)

Tubal problems

If obstruction of the tubes is found by hysterosalpingogram, laparoscopy would help confirm the location and cause of the obstruction. In addition, laparoscopy might uncover unsuspected adhesions around the tubes and/or ovaries or even pelvic endometriosis. In any of these instances, after completion of the other basic portions of the workup your doctor could proceed directly to treatment with no further testing. In fact, many times it is possible to correct these problems at the time of the diagnostic laparoscopy; surgery through the laparoscope (pelviscopy) is becoming a skill many gynecologists are acquiring. Occasionally, the extent of tubal disease may be so clear on the tubal X-ray that in vitro fertilization may be advised even without laparoscopy. In one very specific case, obstruction of the tubes near the uterus, a radiologic technique may be used to directly catheterize the tubes. In many of these cases the tubes may be opened by the procedure, and preliminary results regarding fertility are promising. (RISK—MODERATE; PAIN—LOW TO MODERATE; COST—HIGH)

Cervical factor

If the cervical mucus is full of inflammatory cells, antibiotic treatment is prescribed. If the mucus is poor in quality or quantity, a small dose of preovulatory estrogen may be prescribed. If the PCT shows immobile or shaking sperm, further testing in the form of antisperm antibodies may be performed. In most instances of an abnormal PCT, a trial of four to six intrauterine inseminations is generally recommended. Approximately one third of these patients have been reported to be successful. (RISK—LOW; PAIN—NONE; COST—LOW)

"ALL OF YOUR TESTS ARE NORMAL"

That's what about 5 to 10 percent of patients will hear at the conclusion of this set of tests. They will be categorized as having "unexplained infertility." This does not mean that there is no cause for their infertility problem, only that it has not yet been found. Other tests now need to be done, but there is little or no agreement among infertility specialists as to exactly where these fit into the workup.

Cultures

In couples who are unsuccessful in conceiving without an apparent reason, a variety of tests to determine both common and uncommon causes of infection of the genital tract may be performed at some time during the workup. These may include cultures for chlamydia, a common organism implicated in infertility. A recent study from Italy correlated infertility with a subclinical chlamydial infection in the endometrium of patients who have normal-appearing tubes at laparoscopy. A culture for ureaplasma organisms may be done when there is a history of early pregnancy loss.

For example, Barbara, twenty-eight, and Tom, twenty-eight, came in with a history of eight previous early pregnancy losses. They had been to several doctors; thorough workups had included chromosomal tests to insure that no genetic factor was present. This was some time ago, before the clinical availability of culture methods for ureaplasma. Specimens from Barbara's cervix were sent to one of the research labs testing for this organism. You guessed it! Her culture was positive for ureaplasma. Both she and Tom were treated with a long-acting tetracycline for ten days and then went on to have two healthy children in two successive pregnancies. (RISK—NONE; PAIN—NONE; COST—LOW)

Hormone levels

Certain hormone tests, specifically thyroid function tests and prolactin, may be ordered even if ovulation appears to be normal. Minimal elevations of prolactin can affect the luteal phase of the cycle and cause infertility despite the fact that all other tests are normal. An elevated prolactin suddenly explains "unexplained infertility." Similarly, minimal alterations in thyroid function can also disturb ovulation.

In a small number of patients, correction of an underlying medical problem may lead to pregnancy. Several years ago Janet, twenty-eight, went through the entire workup with all tests normal except for a low normal sperm count on her husband, Michael. When Janet came in complaining of fatigue, a complete medical workup showed slightly high blood sugar. A glucose tolerance test confirmed that she had early diabetes. She was placed on a proper diet and required insulin for adequate control of her blood sugar. When her sugar was controlled she conceived quickly and now has two girls. (RISK—NONE; PAIN—NONE; COST—LOW)

Ultrasound

An uncommon cause of unexplained infertility can be failure of the follicle to rupture at a normal diameter or even rupture entirely (luteinized unruptured follicle—LUF). In order to detect this possibility, a series of vaginal ultrasound examinations can be done to trace the growth of the follicle to a proper peak diameter and its eventual rupture. The ultrasound probe is placed in the vagina and sends sound waves into the tissues which send back an echo creating a picture of the internal organs. When used vaginally, the probe is very close to the pelvic organs and the quality of the image is better than when the probe is placed on the abdomen. Another benefit to the vaginal probe is that there is no need to fill the bladder to capacity, which can be uncomfortable. In order to evaluate follicle dynamics, scans will be done shortly before the anticipated day of ovulation and every one to three days until a normal follicle diameter is reached. The patient will also monitor her LH surge and will return two days following the surge to confirm collapse of the follicle. In one recent study, women with unexplained infertility and a confirmed abnormality of follicle growth and collapse had a very high cumulative pregnancy rate with ovulation induction compared to a rather low rate in women with normal follicle dynamics. (RISK—NONE; PAIN—NONE; COST—LOW TO MODERATE)

Antisperm antibodies

Infertile couples manifest antisperm antibodies in about 15 percent to 20 percent of females and 5 percent to 10 percent in males (as contrasted to about 1 percent to 2 percent of the fertile population). In patients with abnormal mucus penetration the incidence of sperm antibodies is much higher. Of the tests done for immunologic infertility, the immunobead test is thought to be the most specific. In this test, small beads with antibody attached are mixed with sperm. If 10 percent of the sperm bind to the beads the test is considered positive. In couples with a normal postcoital test, these studies are not usually done until late in the workup. In fact, in the face of a normal PCT, many centers do these tests only in anticipation of going on to assisted reproductive procedures or if the sperm in the semen analysis show marked clumping or vibratory movement instead of forward motion. (RISK—NONE; PAIN—NONE; COST—LOW TO MODERATE)

In the usual instance of unexplained infertility, intrauterine insemination (IUI) will be recommended, first with the patient's spontaneous cycle, then with the patient on fertility drugs (see also p. 93). Since IUI is also the treatment for antibodies in either partner, we generally reserve antibody testing until after IUI and before ART. In preparation for the ART cycle, the presence of antibodies may indicate that IVF would maximize fertilization compared with GIFT. And, in some instances of antibodies in the male, a very large number of sperm must be added to the egg for fertilization to occur in vitro.

Fifteen years ago, a much larger proportion of patients would have fallen into the category of unexplained infertility. For those patients we would have had to say "We do not have any specific treatment to offer you. Keep trying. Good-bye and good luck." Today we have a series of what are now considered conventional treatments for the couple with unexplained infertility as well as those in whom we have found an apparent problem. Since a basic principle is to do the safer, simpler, and less expensive treatment first, we'll consider these conventional procedures in Chapter 6 before going on to ART.

six

Honey, It Worked!

Although this is a book about IVF, GIFT, and other types of assisted reproduction, we have spent a good deal of time outlining how the reproductive system works, why it sometimes doesn't work, and how to find out why it doesn't work. We are now about to embark on a discussion of some of the conventional treatments for the various causes of infertility.

There are two reasons we are spending so much time on conventional infertility issues. One reason is that there is no way in the world that anyone could understand the complex issues regarding assisted reproduction without understanding the basics of the human reproductive process along with why and how it can malfunction. After all, in school you can't take Biology 2 until you have completed the necessary prerequisite, Biology 1.

The second reason is to make an important point. We said it before when we were discussing testing. And we say it again here because it is one of the most important points to understand if you are considering ART procedures. You always do the safer, simpler, and less expensive procedures first! In order to make an informed decision regarding your need for the ART procedures, you must be sure that all other reasonable avenues of treatment have been exhausted. Remember, conventional treatment often works.

BASIC MATH

Before we go on to describe the pre-ART infertility treatments, you need to know about the mathematics of reproduction:

RULE 1. Monthly conception rate

For the average "normal" couple without any infertility problem, the chance of conceiving in one cycle—their monthly conception rate—will be between 20 percent and 25 percent if they have intercourse at the proper time of the cycle. This probably represents the maximum efficiency of the human reproductive system. It is important that you keep this in mind as you evaluate success rates of various treatments and your own response to treatment. For example, if a treatment is recommended and it does not work the first month, don't be discouraged. Even if it did totally correct your problem, according to this rule you still have only a maximum 20-to-25-percent chance of getting pregnant that first month. Many couples who do not understand this get discouraged and consequently give up before they have given a specific treatment an adequate chance.

RULE 2. Cumulative conception rate

The next logical step is that you must also look at the success of a treatment from the viewpoint of time. If in our "normal" couple we tried to calculate the chance of getting pregnant, it would naturally depend on how long they tried. If they tried for only one month, their conception rate would be, let's say, 20 percent. Yet you cannot say that this couple has only a 20 percent chance of getting pregnant. Let us go further out in time and look at a hundred "normal" couples. After one month twenty couples would have gotten pregnant, eighty would still not have conceived. In the second month, sixteen would conceive (20 percent of eighty couples) and sixty-four would be left not pregnant:

Month	# Couples left	# Pregnant	# Not Pregnant
1	100	20	80
2	80	16	64
3	64	13	51
4	51	10	41
5	41	8	33
6	33	7	26
7	26	5	21

Month	# Couples left	# Pregnant	# Not Pregnant
8	21	4	17
9	17	3	14
10	14	3	11
11	11	2	9
12	9	2	7

So the cumulative conception rate in this group of "normal" patients should be 93 percent in twelve cycles. In fact, the true pattern does not strictly follow this rule, because all woman are not the same. Included in these hundred women will be some who are highly fertile and some who have inherent low fertility or even a specific infertility problem. Actually, about 80 percent of couples attempting pregnancy will conceive within one year.

Using this cumulative rate, you can see how we can arrive at the time interval of one year as significant in defining infertility. If you have been trying for only six months, there is still a 26 percent chance you would not have conceived even if you were "normal." Since as many as 26 percent of normal couples would not conceive by six months, it does not pay to begin a workup at that time unless there are extenuating circumstances, such as age or a recognized infertility factor.

The cumulative conception rate is also important to keep in mind if you are planning to go through an ART procedure because the implication of this rule is that in order to achieve the maximum chance of success, you will have to consider going through several cycles. If a program has, for instance, a 20 percent "take-home baby rate" and you go through one cycle, you have a 20 percent chance. There is no single factor more important to a final successful outcome than having repeated cycles. We've said it before: Persistence is the key ingredient of success.

RULE 3. *Your* conception rate

You need to think of your infertility problem in terms of what it does to your monthly conception rate. You can then estimate how a particular treatment will modify your monthly rate and project it to a cumulative conception rate. This will give you an idea of how long you may wish to try a specific treatment.

Let's say your problem is azoospermia and you have decided to use donor sperm to overcome the problem. You can assume that the monthly conception rate with donor sperm is about 15 percent. You could calculate the cumulative rate as follows:

Month	# Couples	# Pregnant	# Not pregnant
1	100	15	85
2	85	13	72
3	72	11	61
4	61	9	52
5	52	8	44
6	44	7	37
7	37	6	31
8	31	5	26
9	26	4	22
10	18	3	15
11	15	2	13
12	13	2	11

By one year of artificial insemination all but 11 percent of otherwise normal women would be pregnant by donor insemination. Again, it is not actually this high because some of the women will have other fertility problems. So, if you are not pregnant by this time, it might be safe to assume that there may be an additional factor over and above the azoospermia, and further tests would be indicated. This would probably not be true after six months, when 37 percent of otherwise normal women would not have conceived. And it certainly does not make sense to stop after only three months of donor insemination because, at that point, we know there is a 61 percent chance that you would not be successful. It would be too soon to stop.

We can't say it too often: Perseverance pays off! Now you know how to figure out how long to persevere.

RULE 4.   The exception to the rule

This is a modification of Rule 3. As you go further out in time, the pregnancy rate does not always approach 100 percent and the not-pregnant rate 0 percent, since our treatments are not perfect. There are often periods of time after which no pregnancies occur. For example, if we treat endometriosis with surgery, most of the pregnancies occur in the first year. From one to three years there is a decrease in the monthly conception rate, and after three years virtually no pregnancies occur. This can happen either because scarring from the endometriosis may have recurred following surgery or the couple may have, at this point, other factors for which they may need further evaluation and treatment.

Monthly and cumulative pregnancy rates for most infertility factors and treatments have been worked out and published. Success rates of new developments are often reported in this fashion too, so this information can be obtained.

HOW SUCCESSFUL IS TREATMENT?

That large 1980 study cited in Chapter 5 not only discussed the causes of infertility in its patient population but also related the cause to actual results of treatment. One of the most interesting aspects of the study projected what the success rate should have been based on the cumulative conception rate for that particular condition *if* the patients had continued treatment indefinitely:

| | Pregnancy rate | |
	Actual Percent	Expected Percent
Endometriosis	31	52
Male factor	38	74
Lack of ovulation	44	79
Tubal factor	26	48
Luteal phase problems	46	58
Cervical factor	26	45
Uterine factor	33	38

Remember, the rates for most of these are better today than they were before 1980, due largely to better conventional treatments and the advent of assisted reproduction.

The fact that the expected rates are much higher than the actual rates makes one of our most important points: Many people give up too early! That is not to say that you should try a particular treatment indefinitely. You should, along with your doctor, be able to rationally determine how long to pursue any and all treatment, using the concept of cumulative conception rates. It's like what they say about the stock market: many experts know when to buy a stock, but few know when to sell. Or, as Kenny Rogers advises in his song, "The Gambler," you've got to "know when to hold 'em, know when to fold 'em." In infertility, there is usually good rationale for the selection of a particular treatment, but few guidelines on how long to persist. It takes a lot of experience to know when to hold 'em and when to fold 'em.

SPECIFIC TREATMENT

Lack of ovulation

Most treatment for anovulation falls into one of three regimens:
- Clomiphene citrate (CC)
- Human menopausal gonadotrophins (hMG) with or without clomiphene
- Gonadotropin-releasing hormone (GnRH)

Exceptions to use of these drugs would be in patients with documented hormone problems which can be overcome by the administration of a specific hormone to correct the problem. Patients falling in this category would include those with an elevated prolactin level with or without galactorrhea or evidence of a microadenoma of the pituitary gland. These people will be treated specifically with bromocriptine (Parlodel), which will reduce the level of prolactin, eliminate the galactorrhea, shrink the microadenoma, and allow ovulation to return to normal.

Bromocriptine is taken orally. It is relatively inexpensive and significant side effects are infrequent. The dose is usually increased gradually based on the reduction in prolactin. It takes from four to six weeks to relieve the galactorrhea, reduce serum prolactin, and resume menses. The success rate is fairly high, with about 80 percent of patients responding with ovulation and over 60 percent becoming pregnant. Cost averages about $1.25 a tablet, or $75 for a month's therapy at two tablets a day.

Another example of the use of a specific medication occurs in women who may have symptoms of excessive hair growth, acne, and lack of a menstrual cycle due to excessive adrenal hormones. These women can be treated specifically with a cortisonelike drug such as dexamethasone, usually taken at bedtime. Again, this treatment is specific, effective, relatively inexpensive, and free of side effects with short-term treatment. A third example involves women who are low in thyroid hormone and whose lack of ovulation can be corrected with simple and inexpensive thyroid hormone pills.

But the vast majority of patients with ovulatory problems will be treated with the three major drugs.

CLOMIPHENE CITRATE (CC—SEROPHENE, CLOMID). The first drug available for ovulation induction was discovered by accident. It is an antiestrogen and was being studied as a contraceptive agent designed to block the implantation process in animals. When it was applied to humans it was noticed that it increased gonadotropins and caused ovulation. For over twenty-five years it has been used as the first-line drug for the induction of ovulation.

Clomiphene is used in patients whose ovulatory problem is caused by a malfunction in the hypothalamus (due to the causes discussed in Chapter 4) and in patients with polycystic ovaries/Stein-Leventhal syndrome. On a practical basis, clomiphene is often tried first in patients who are producing adequate amounts of estrogen because it is relatively inexpensive, easy to monitor, and readily available to all physicians. It is taken orally, starting the third to fifth day of the cycle. A pelvic examination or ultrasound is usually done prior to starting treatment to make sure that no ovarian cysts are present. The drug is usually taken for five days and, if ovulation does not occur, the dose increased in succeeding cycles.

As infertility treatments go, the cost of clomiphene is modest. Retail cost can vary but is around $4 to $7 a tablet. You may want to inquire from the pharmacist which brand he or she is giving you and compare the costs of each, since Clomid and Serophene are pharmaceutically equivalent. Side effects are not usually a problem but may consist of enlargement of the ovaries and/or abdominal discomfort. Risks include:

- Multiple pregnancy in about 8 percent of patients (most often twins)
- Development of ovarian cysts
- Overstimulation of the ovaries in a very small number of patients

Overstimulation is a potentially serious problem causing an imbalance in the body's fluids and electrolytes (discussed in the section on hMG therapy, below). Minor side effects include hot flushes, breast tenderness, headache, nervousness, dizziness, nausea and vomiting, and fatigue. In addition, it can also rarely cause visual disturbances that should be reported to your doctor. In our experience, most patients on clomiphene feel perfectly fine. There is no evidence that clomiphene causes birth defects when used for induction of ovulation.

Success rates vary tremendously from study to study and range between 30 percent to 90 percent. In general, about 50 percent to 90 percent of women with abnormal menstrual cycles will achieve ovulation with clomiphene and about half of those will get pregnant if given an adequate trial. If all other factors are normal, the conception rate for clomiphene-induced ovulation should approach those of cycles in which ovulation occurred spontaneously. Failure to achieve pregnancy after successful ovulation with clomiphene may be due to any of the following factors:

- An unwanted effect from the clomiphene such as decrease in cervical mucus or poor endometrial development
- Poor-quality eggs because the hormonal environment of the ovary is not normal
- Other causes of infertility that may be present
- Lack of persistence. In one study of patients with no other fertility factors, the pregnancy rate approached 100 percent when corrected for the 44 percent of patients who dropped out before completing enough cycles.

Your cycle will likely be monitored with a basal body temperature chart and/or urinary LH testing. Some physicians will check a serum progesterone level during the luteal phase to check its adequacy. With some patients who do not ovulate, physicians may add a shot of HCG (a pregnancy hormone that simulates the LH surge) about eight days after the clomiphene is finished. Some choose to follow the follicle development via vaginal ultrasound and then administer HCG when the follicle reaches mature size. Ultrasound done two days later can assure that the follicle has actually ruptured.

The majority of pregnancies occur within the first four to six cycles of treatment. This is based on a monthly conception rate estimated by one group as 22 percent if no other fertility factors were present, which does not really differ from normal couples. This group of physicians felt that the rate declined after ten months of therapy. Now you can construct your own table to determine how long you should stick with this treatment.

Human Menopaural Gonadotropin (hMG—Pergonal). Consisting of both FSH and LH, hMG is generally used in patients who do not produce their own gonadotropins and secrete inadequate amounts of estrogen. It is also helpful in those patients who do not respond to clomiphene. In the late 1950s and early 1960s gonadotropins were first extracted from the urine of menopausal women in Italy, and it was not long before they were tried for ovulation induction. There were major problems from the start because the tools for monitoring its use were rudimentary and the multiple pregnancy rate was high. At first, doctors monitored their patients with pelvic examination, vaginal smears for estrogen level, observation of the cervical mucus, and urinary estrogen determinations. Monitoring has vastly improved, first with the advent of the rapid urinary estrogen test, now with the rapid serum estrogen test by radioimmunoassay and pelvic ultrasound. Recently, the use of vaginal ultrasound probes has made monitoring more comfortable and even more accurate. More precise monitoring of hMG cycles has resulted in a reduction of the multiple-pregnancy rate from 28 percent to less than 10 percent and the almost complete absence of high-order multiple pregnancies (four or more babies). Patients considering hMG therapy should be aware, however, that although ultrasound monitoring reduces the risk, it is not absolute. Generally, follicles above 14 to 16 millimeters mean diameter are considered mature and capable of ovulation. However, follicles below this size can sometimes result in pregnancy. Just as with IVF, some surprisingly small follicles can yield mature eggs. Before you accept hMG therapy, be sure that you will be adequately monitored by a vaginal ultrasound and measurement of one of the estrogens, estradiol. While some obstetricians and gynecologists have the facilities to do this, others don't.

Because of the high cost of hMG and its side effects, efforts should first be made to achieve pregnancy by simpler means. Currently the retail cost of one vial of hMG is about $44. With fifteen or more vials possibly necessary to complete the cycle the cost of medication exceeds $660 for one cycle. Add to that three or four pelvic ultrasounds and a rapid serum estradiol and you are likely to spend over $1000 on one cycle of treatment. This has led some physicians to use a combination of clomiphene and hMG (CC/hMG) that requires less hMG, thus cutting costs somewhat.

It also leads patients to look for ways of cutting costs. We recently encountered a patient on hMG therapy for anovulation who needed more than one vial per day to stimulate adequate follicles. We were reluctant to go to two vials because we wanted to avoid multiple pregnancy as she had been exposed to DES and had a small T-shaped uterus. Giving her one and one half a day would be wasteful because half a vial would be unusable. She said she didn't care. When she felt that she might need this treatment, she convinced her employer to offer a "drug card" with their health plan and all she paid was $5 for her entire supply of hMG.

There are many different ways of prescribing hMG, but most physicians start at a dose of one to two vials a day, starting on the second to fifth day of the cycle. The patient is then seen again after four to seven days of injections, at which time the response may be assessed by ultrasound and/or checking estradiol levels. The dose is adjusted, and the patient returns in one to three days, depending on the number and size of her follicles. When the follicles reach mature size in an acceptable number (one to three), the serum estradiol may be checked and the HCG is given to simulate the LH surge, triggering ovulation. Ovulation should occur about thirty-six to forty-four hours after the HCG. The patient is instructed to have intercourse accordingly, or in some cases she will have insemination, depending if other problems such as a male factor may be present.

The risks of hMG are similar to, but considerably more significant than, those of clomiphene. Side effects may include ovarian cysts, abdominal distention and pain, multiple pregnancy, and ovarian hyperstimulation. Most of these do not progress and will usually resolve if the hMG is stopped, HCG is not given, and the patient does not become pregnant. Overstimulation can be mild, with fluid retention, enlarged ovaries, and abdominal discomfort. When severe, significant fluid imbalance may require hospitalization. Other side effects include allergy to hMG, pain, rash, swelling, and irritation at the injection site. Mood swings may occur while on the medication. In addition, you may notice an increased amount of cervical mucus because of the increased amounts of estrogen. Overall, the incidence of birth defects in patients using hMG to induce ovulation is not any higher than that of the general population.

A new twist to the use of gonadotropins has been the development of pure FSH (Metrodin). It is administered and monitored in the same manner as hMG and, may be used in combination with hMG. The benefit to certain patients is that pure FSH has practically no LH in it and therefore it may be an advantage to patients who have an elevated level of LH. Patients with polycystic ovaries and an elevated LH fall into this category. If we give more LH, it can stimulate the production of certain hormones called androgens, and these can interfere with development or health of the follicle. Studies of the circulating levels of LH and FSH after injection of the two drugs has shown higher levels of FSH and lower levels of LH with metrodin.

GONADOTROPIN-RELEASING HORMONE (GNRH PUMP). Relatively new on the market, its use has been studied in women with a wide variety of causes for their anovulation. It is highly effective in hypothalamic amenorrhea, less effective in PCO. The main requirement has been that the patient must have normal pituitary function, although recent studies show it is effective in higher-than-usual doses if the pituitary is impaired. Like hMG and pure FSH, it must be given by injection, but its action is completely different. Instead of being a gonadotropin, it stimulates the pituitary to secrete its own gonadotropins in normal sequence. It actually simulates a normal cycle. Therefore, as you would expect, you avoid the greater chance of multiple pregnancy and overstimulation associated with hMG.

The catch is that GnRH must be administered in pulses, usually every ninety minutes. Since it is impractical to take injections every ninety minutes around the clock, it is administered by an automatic pump worn around the waist with a needle inserted under the skin or into a vein. The cycle is monitored by vaginal ultrasound every few days to document the growth and collapse of the follicle. The pump is disconnected after ovulation is verified and then HCG is given to support the corpus luteum.

Except for some tissue reaction at the needle site, there are no serious side effects or complications. Data regarding effectiveness is optimistic, showing fairly high ovulation and success rates (about 30 per ovulatory cycle), but number of cases is small. The cost for one cycle of treatment would be in the neighborhood of about $600.

Unfortunately, there are causes of lack of ovulation and menses that are not treatable with these measures. But causes such as chromosomal defects, premature ovarian failure, and surgical removal of the ovaries are now treatable with the use of donor eggs through IVF techniques (discussed in Chapter 11).

Claire, in her early twenties, is a good example of the type of expense and difficulty some patients with significant ovulatory problems must endure. She was diagnosed as having Kallman's syndrome, a combination of lack of ovulation because of low gonadotropins and loss of the sense of smell. This can be very difficult to treat, but it responds well to the GnRH pump. When she started treatment, the pump was not available. She went through six cycles of hMG–HCG without getting pregnant, using up to sixty ampules of hMG each cycle, costing over $2,000 per cycle for medication alone. When the GnRH pump was available, she conceived on her first try.

Male factor

When you consider that a fairly large proportion of infertility is due to the male factor, it is surprising that the treatment of the male factor has been largely ignored until recently. Nearly twenty years ago, all we could offer the couple with a significant male factor infertility was artificial insemination with semen from a donor, artificial insemination with the husband's semen, or repair of a varicocele.

During the last decade, we've seen a great deal of interest in the workup and treatment of the male. This interest has paralleled advances in ART and the need to prepare the sperm for these advanced techniques. It bears repeating that changes in habits, when possible, should be recommended first to try to maximize the couple's chances of conceiving. For the male partner these would include changes in sexual frequency and timing; eliminating heated spa-type baths; changing from briefs to boxer shorts; and avoiding drugs, smoking, and exposure to toxins.

Again, just as we categorized conditions causing male infertility according to the results of the semen analysis, we can break down treatment into the same categories.

NORMAL SEMEN ANALYSIS. If the female's evaluation and the initial semen analyses were normal, the man may be tested with more sophisticated tests of sperm function such as computer-assisted semen analysis and sperm penetration assay (SPA—hamster test) in which the ability of his sperm to penetrate a hamster egg with the zona removed will be evaluated. Just as with other male factors, pregnancy may be possible with intrauterine insemination or IVF, sometimes by modifying the way in which sperm are prepared.

AZOOSPERMIA. In the complete absence of sperm, a hormone workup will help reveal the nature of the problem. If the man's gonadotropins

(FSH and LH) are very high, it can be assumed that he has testicular failure. The only treatment now available is artificial insemination with the semen of a donor. If the couple is unwilling to have donor insemination, they could consider adoption.

If his gonadotropins are normal or slightly elevated, he may have an obstruction of the ductal system and should have an operation called a scrotal exploration to determine the location of the obstruction and attempt to correct it. This is major surgery, with all of its risks, at a cost of about $3,000 to $6,000. It is an outpatient surgery procedure usually performed under general anesthesia. The variation in cost will generally reflect the complexity of the repair and the time required to perform the operation, from one and a half to five hours. Before the scrotal exploration, the urologist may recommend a biopsy of the testicle as a separate procedure to determine if enough sperm are present before proceeding on to the more serious scrotal exploration. The biopsy is also an outpatient procedure that can be performed under either local or general anesthesia at a cost of about $1,000.

In cases of congenital absence of portions of the tubular system, microsurgical procedures are now being used to retrieve sperm directly from the epididymis for use in conjunction with ART procedures.

In the face of low gonadotropins with low testosterone levels and the presence of the sugar fructose in the semen, the man would need further evaluation of his pituitary hormones. Fructose is produced by the seminal vesicles, and its presence in the semen makes blockage of the tubular system unlikely. As in the woman, if his prolactin is significantly elevated with or without evidence of a pituitary microadenoma, he would be treated with bromocriptine. If his gonadotropins are low, he can be treated with HCG and hMG.

A special category of obstruction is the case of a man who has had a vasectomy and wants it reversed. This can be accomplished by microscopic surgery or laser-assisted microsurgery. In addition to the area of the vasectomy's intentional blockage, other areas of obstruction may develop in adjacent locations and must be searched for and bypassed. In general, the success of vasovasostomy will be related to the length of time that has elapsed between the vasectomy and its repair and the skill and experience of the surgeon performing the procedure.

OTHER ABNORMALITIES. Here one of the conditions the physician may suspect is a varicocele. If one is found, it should be corrected after other nonsurgical problems, such as hormonal or environmental causes, have been looked for and corrected. If no varicocele is present, many physicians will try to stimulate better sperm production with hormones, usually clomiphene or HCG. Recent studies have shown that a very small dose of clomiphene stimulates increased output of active sperm.

The role of surgery to try to overcome infertility by correcting a varicocele is controversial. Of course, our basic premise applies here: that the simple, safe, and less expensive treatments must be explored first. Therefore, in the face of consistently abnormal semen analyses and normal tests of pituitary function, other causes of the abnormal semen must be considered: chronic use of drugs, infection, physical stress, and exposure to toxic agents such as X-rays, pesticides, industrial chemicals, or heat. Then if there are no other apparent causes for the abnormal semen analysis or there are other abnormal tests of sperm function, a varicocele should be searched for and surgery should be considered.

Special tests such as a venogram to help verify the presence of a varicocele are sometimes necessary and can be conducted on an outpatient basis. The varicocele is repaired through a 1.5-inch incision in the groin. Thus the veins are blocked above the testicle. This blockage of the flow of blood from the testicle does not cause damage because there are two other vein systems leaving the testicle. The discomfort after surgery is moderate and can be managed with oral pain medication. Most men can go back to work in three to four days and resume strenuous activity in three to four weeks.

Improvement in the semen analysis or fertility cannot be expected for at least three months. In properly selected men there will be a 60 percent to 70 percent chance for improvement in the semen analysis, but possibly not until up to one year after surgery. The pregnancy rate reaches 40 percent to 45 percent while men not treated have rates in the range of 15 percent to 20 percent. So, at best, varicocelectomy can provide a two-to-three-times improvement in pregnancy rates. An alternative to surgery would be ART procedures. But most urologists would recommend varicocelectomy in the case of an obvious varicocele with indications of abnormal semen and especially if the affected testicle is smaller than its mate. With all treatments of the female, including ART procedures, the chance of success will be better with the male factor improved as much as possible.

If the semen analysis reveals decreased motility, sperm antibodies may be searched for, especially if the sperm are seen to clump together. If antibodies are found, then high doses of steroids may be prescribed for short periods to avoid the long-term side effects. Finally, the husband's sperm can be used for artificial insemination into the uterus after washing (AIH-IUI), as is commonly done for cervical mucus problems.

Small volume or the complete absence of semen can occur as the result of retrograde ejaculation, or ejaculation backward into the bladder. If the retrograde ejaculation is due to medical conditions such as diabetes, semen can be obtained by use of drugs that close the bladder neck. If retrograde ejaculation is the result of a complication of previous surgery, sperm can be harvested from a urine specimen (after masturbation) and then prepared for artificial insemination. If the specimen is voided into culture medium and the acidity of the urine is adjusted by taking baking soda, the sperm will survive for a brief period of time in the urine. In some instances it is necessary to adjust the concentration of the urine.

Endometriosis

The treatment of endometriosis can fall into two general categories— medical and surgical. In fact, also now emerging is a third category— no treatment. This is because an accumulating body of evidence indicates that infertility patients with minimal to mild stages of endometriosis who undergo no treatment may have the same conception rate as those treated by medications or surgery. Actually, endometriosis treatment is very complex and dependent on symptoms, location, and degree of the disease. (Its thorough consideration is beyond the scope of this book.)

At issue currently is whether it is necessary to treat endometriosis in an infertile woman when the degree of the disease is minimal. The pregnancy rate resulting from no treatment (31 percent to 75 percent over eighteen months) is very similar to the rate when operative or medical treatment is used. The issue of "no treatment" is somewhat moot, however, because when laparoscopy is done to make the diagnosis, the implants can easily be cauterized or lasered through the laparoscope, thus preventing progression of the disease. If your endometriosis is minimal and it was not treated at the time of laparoscopy, you may want to try to conceive without going through a course of medical therapy that may not be necessary.

Medical treatment

The first hormonal treatment for endometriosis was based on the fact that pregnancy seemed to have the effect of improving endometriosis. Physicians thus tried to create a pseudopregnancy state with the use of hormones. This was accomplished by using either synthetic progesteronelike compounds (progestins) or birth control pills. The birth control pills are still used for this purpose, although newer drugs are now available and are more effective.

BIRTH CONTROL PILLS. In the early days of hormonal treatment, continuous use of the birth control pill was popular because it was safe, effective, convenient, and inexpensive. Since the subsequent pregnancy rate was fairly low (15 percent to 30 percent), other medications were developed and are now used more frequently. The patient can be started on one birth control pill per day, but instead of stopping the pill after three weeks, it is continued for a total of nine months. If the patient develops bleeding while on this regimen, the dose of the pill may be gradually increased. It has been thought that patients should not have any menstrual periods while on this treatment. This will allow the areas of endometriosis to subside. The use of the pill is relatively safe, although increasing to higher doses will increase the risk of blood clots and other complications of oral contraceptives. Common but minor side effects include nausea, breast tenderness, headaches, irritability, fluid retention, and spotting. One advantage of the pill is its low cost. A month of continuous therapy should cost less than $20.

PROGESTINS. If a woman is unwilling to take birth control pills or should not because of previous problems with blood clots, she may be put on a progestin, one of the synthetic compounds that have action similar to progesterone. A common one used is medroxyprogesterone acetate. It can be given as daily pills (Provera, Amen, Curretab) or as a long-acting injection (Depo-Provera). It is a fairly innocuous medication as far as side effects are concerned and cost is fairly low. We do not feel that the long-acting injection should be given to infertility patients because it can cause prolonged amenorrhea. It is best to fully suppress the disease, then try to conceive without delay.

There has been a great deal of attention in the media about studies relating long-term progestin therapy to breast cancer, especially in postmenopausal women. These findings are highly controversial and should not be of concern since they have not been found with continuous use of progestins and use for endometriosis for short periods.

DANAZOL (DANOCRINE). This is now a very popular method of hormonal suppression of endometriosis. Danazol acts to supress the ovary and create a kind of pseudo-menopausal state. However, the fact that it is related in structure to the male hormone testosterone accounts for most of its side effects. These can include unwanted hair growth on the face and body, acne, deepening of the voice, weight gain, decreased breast size as well as amenorrhea or abnormal bleeding. It also may have a detrimental effect by reducing "good" cholesterol. In addition, the drug is costly, averaging about $200 for a month's treatment at the maximum dose. The pregnancy rate (30 to 60 percent) is higher than with the pill.

GONADOTROPIN-RELEASING HORMONE (GNRH) AGONISTS. Potent long-acting forms of GnRH (agonists) such as leuprolide (Lupron) are given by daily injection. They initially stimulate gonadotropins, but as they are continued they supress the pituitary. The resulting reduction of gonadotropins causes the ovary to almost cease its production of estrogen. Since endometrium is dependent on estrogen for continued growth, the endometriosis shrinks. Pregnancy rates are similar to results using danazol. Its side effects are related to a lack of estrogen and include hot flushes, vaginal dryness, decreased libido, and even some bone loss. Unlike danazol, it does not appear to have a detrimental effect on the favorable type of cholesterol.

There is now a long-acting form of the medication on the market (Lupron DEPOT), which is given every four weeks. Most women are adequately suppressed at half the dose, allowing two women to be treated with each receiving half of one vial, thus limiting cost. Leuprolide is currently not FDA-approved for treating endometriosis.

Nevertheless, physicians use it widely for this purpose. It is a common practice for physicians to use approved drugs for nonapproved indications when it will benefit their patients.

Other GnRH agonists being investigated are nafarelin (Synarel) and buserelin. These have the advantage of not requiring injections since they are administered as a nasal spray. Synarel was approved in January 1990 for the management of endometriosis, pelvic pain caused by endometriosis, and treatment of endometriosis lesions. Although Synarel is not specifically approved for treating infertility, treatment of the endometriosis could result in improved fertility, as with other medical and surgical treatments.

SURGICAL TREATMENT. Surgical options for endometriosis include either laparoscopy or open surgery through a conventional incision. The current trend is for more aggressive use of the laparoscope utilizing electrocautery, various lasers, and other surgical techniques (pelviscopy) through the scope to destroy areas of endometriosis (implants), remove cysts, break up adhesions, and even remove tubes and ovaries when necessary. The advantage of laparoscopy over conventional surgery is that it is done through very small incisions, can be an outpatient procedure, requires less recuperation, and is less costly.

Many times very adequate treatment of even unsuspected endometriosis can be done at the time of an initial diagnostic laparoscopy. Before submitting to the initial diagnostic laparoscopy, it might be a good idea to ask if the surgeon is experienced and prepared to treat any conditions found at that time. In general, substantial amounts of endometriosis can be dealt with adequately through the scope. More severe degrees of endometriosis may require an operation through a conventional incision. In addition, the combination of endometriosis with other abnormalities such as tubal problems or fibroids needing removal might require open surgery, although even tubal obstruction can sometimes be treated through the laparoscope.

The conception rates following laser treatment of endometrial implants (50 percent to 73 percent) is slightly better than those reported using electrocautery (50 percent to 60 percent), but many authorities feel that the apparent slight difference in rates is not significant. Just be sure that your doctor feels comfortable handling mild to moderate degrees of endometriosis through the laparoscope so you won't be subjected to needless additional surgery or medical therapy.

Following surgery, hormonal treatment may be considered. In some cases, postoperative medical therapy together with laparoscopic surgery is advisable.

Tubal Problems

The most important recent advances in tubal surgery have been the use of microsurgical techniques: the operating microscope, small sutures, microsurgical instruments, and new tissue-handling techniques to reduce the risk of postoperative adhesions. The laser has been used in tubal infertility surgery even more recently, but its use is still controversial. Although many infertility surgeons advocate it and find that it saves time and facilitates certain aspects of tubal repair, there is no solid evidence that success rates are improved by the use of the laser. Newer "superpulse" modes of the laser reduce tissue injury by about half and may mean a significant improvement over standard continuous beams. Also, new methods are becoming available for prevention of postoperative adhesions, such as the recently released peritoneal patches (Interceed).

Before we discuss success rates with surgery, you must realize that relatively few surgeons have enough personal experience to be able to quote meaningful success rates based on *their own* experience. Here is an opportunity for you to be a good consumer. Find someone in your community with a prominent reputation for *this type* of surgery. Generally, such an individual will have done at least a hundred microsurgical cases and does them on a fairly regular basis. The rates quoted below assume you have found a highly experienced surgeon.

The chance of success depends on the type of disease being treated:
- The best pregnancy rates occur when surgery is done purely to correct adhesions (lysis of adhesions) with essentially normal tubes. These adhesions can range from mild to severe. Surgery to remove adhesions will result in a 50 percent to 70 percent conception rate, with the better rate occurring when the adhesions are mild.
- If the blockage in the tube is close to the uterus and the damaged area can be removed with the remaining ends put together (anastamosis), success rates will also be in the range of 50 percent to 70 percent.

Newer methods are being used to catheterize and reopen this type of obstruction without surgery, and preliminary results are encouraging regarding pregnancy.

- When the damage involves the fimbriated end of the tube but the tube is open, plastic surgery to reconstruct the fimbria (fimbrioplasty) yields average conception rates of 40 percent to 60 percent.
- If the tube is closed at the fimbriated end and has be opened (salpingostomy) and then repaired, the results are relatively poor. You can expect a success rate of 10 percent to 40 percent. If the tube, in addition to being closed, has developed into a large hydrosalpinx, the pregnancy rates are even worse, averaging 5 percent to 10 percent.
- A totally separate category consists of women who have had their tubes "tied" and who later decide they want to become pregnant. Depending on the method used to "tie" the tubes, the results of techniques to reverse sterilization can vary from good to poor.

The first step in the process is to determine how the tubes were "tied." If it was performed by placing a clip or Falope ring through the laparoscope or by tying with a suture, the outlook for success would be good (80 percent to 90 percent). Electrocautery using a bipolar instrument would yield fair results, while cautery using the older unipolar technique destroys more of the tube, reducing results further (50 percent to 60 percent). Additionally, repair of an older tubal ligation in which the fimbria was removed (fibriectomy) is even lower (40 percent to 50 percent).

If cautery was used, a laparoscopy should be done to see if there is enough tube left to anticipate good results. It is generally recognized that at least 4 centimeters of the normally 10- to 12-centimeter tube is required to expect a reasonable chance of success. In summary, you can expect:

	Percent
Clip or Falope ring	90
Ligation with suture	80
Bipolar cautery	70
Unipolar cautery	60
Fimbriectomy repair	40

This leads us to the logical conclusion that, with the advent of IVF and with the success rates of some centers in the mid-20-percent range, the surgical procedures that do not yield pregnancy rates above

30 percent to 50 percent should be discouraged and the patient should be counseled to consider IVF. The cost of a major tubal repair would usually be in the range of $12,000, including doctor, assistant, anesthesia, and hospital and run the risks of major surgery and require many weeks of recuperation. If a couple is willing to commit to several cycles of IVF in a center with a 20 percent "take-home" pregnancy rate, their cumulative success rate would be 20 percent after one cycle, 36 percent after two cycles, and 51 percent after three cycles. The major surgery and recuperation are avoided and the cost may be similar. One of the factors in the cost is the availability of insurance, but at present most insurance plans cover neither the surgery nor IVF. If a tubal repair works, you get a bargain in that if it works a second time, it is at no extra cost.

The decision of whether to have surgery or IVF can be complex. The following table puts all of the variables into perspective. Faced

	SURGERY	IVF
TYPE OF PROCEDURE	major incision 4–6 week recovery	nonsurgical minimal recovery
SUCCESS RATE	5% to 90% depending on nature of disease, surgeon	5% to 25% depending on center
ANOTHER PREGNANCY	possible	further cycle and expense
TUBAL PREGNANCY	5 to 25% of pregnancies[a]	1% to 10% of pregnancies depending on problem
MULTIPLE PREGNANCY	1%	up to 40% depending on center[b]
TIME TO PREGNANCY	up to 5 years[c]	1 to several months
INSURANCE	?	?
COST	$12,000	$6000

[a]Rates for tubal pregnancy are often quoted per patient, but only a percentage of patients become pregnant, so the proportion of pregnancies that are ectopic is much higher. With reversal of tubal ligation it is less than 5%, but with badly damaged tubes, it could be over 25%.

[b]The multiple pregnancy rate in a particular center rises in parallel with the success rate. Consequently the better centers usually transfer fewer embryos.

[c]Pregnancies after surgery can occur the next month or over as long as five years or more. A couple should generally wait at least two years following surgery before going on to an ART procedure, although a shorter period of time could be reasonable if more than one pregnancy is desired or if the couple is older.

with the same factors, different couples may reach different conclusions based on which factors may be important to them. For example, if the nearest IVF center is four hours away, it may be better to travel once for tubal surgery, since the IVF cycle requires several visits.

Luteal phase defect (LPD)

There is much discussion among infertility specialists regarding diagnosis and treatment of luteal phase defects, despite the fact that this problem does not occur very often. Treatment is designed to give the luteal phase a hormonal boost to bring it to the appropriate length if it is too short or mature the endometrium at the proper rate if it is lagging behind where it should be. This can be done in any one of several ways.

Since there may be a deficiency in the production of progesterone, the doctor can simply administer progesterone by daily injection, or twice-daily progesterone vaginal suppositories. This would be continued from just after ovulation until the results of a pregnancy test two weeks after ovulation. If the pregnancy test is positive, the progesterone is continued, usually as suppositories. If it is negative, the progesterone is stopped and the menstrual period will occur. Both the injections and suppositories are fairly inexpensive and relatively free of side effects. Remember, the progesterone itself could cause a delay in your period, so the lack of a period while you are on the progesterone does not necessarily mean that you are pregnant.

Another approach is the use of clomiphene to improve an inadequate luteal phase. It is taken in the same manner as in patients who are not ovulating. One paradoxical aspect is that the use of clomiphene itself can result in an inadequate luteal phase.

Small doses of HCG have also been employed on the third, sixth, and ninth days following ovulation to treat this problem. This is generally only done when LPD occurs during ovulation induction. Again, this is inexpensive, free from side effects, and effective. In fact, some centers are routinely using HCG in this manner in patients on hMG to boost the luteal phase to counteract the effects of the high levels of estrogen that result from the production of multiple follicles.

Neither progesterone nor clomiphene has been highly effective. Recent research points out that patients with LPD appear to be of two types:

- Those with poor development of the follicle. Progesterone won't help if the egg is not normal or is not being released.
- Those with normal follicle development, but simply too little progesterone.

The first group appears to do better with clomiphene to develop a normal follicle that will then produce higher levels of progesterone after ovulation. The second group needs only progesterone. Clomiphene may actually do harm to the second group by blocking adequate estrogen development of the endometrium necessary to prepare it to respond to progesterone. It is recommended that a biopsy be done to confirm that the defect has been corrected. If the endometrium remains abnormal after treatment, pregnancies occur infrequently and usually miscarry.

Vivian, thirty-two, was a runner before she started trying to conceive. Although told that this could result in lower luteal phase progestrone levels, she was an avid runner and did not want to stop. Two endometrial biopsies showed a consistent defect, but on ultrasound her follicles behaved normally. A repeat biopsy after treatment with progesterone suppositories confirmed correction of the defect and she became pregnant in the third cycle of treatment and delivered a healthy girl. She now runs while pushing a stroller!

Cervical Problems

Recently, one of the more popular infertility treatments has been intrauterine insemination (IUI) with washed sperm. Previous treatments, including antibiotics to decrease inflammation, estrogen to improve mucus production, and insemination into the cervical mucus were not very effective. Placing the sperm in the uterus bypasses the mucus and eliminates the cervical problem as a factor. It is known to be useful in the treatment of poor quality mucus or mucus that has antibodies which clump and immobilize sperm. As mentioned, this technique is also successful for mild to moderate reductions of semen quality.

Although the chance of success varies with the individual problem, IUI yields about a 30 percent conception rate over three to six cycles, or 5 percent to 10 percent per cycle. In such couples the monthly conception rate without treatment might be 1 percent to 3 percent. It is entirely possible that this treatment "telescopes" successes into the treatment cycle which may have occurred spontaneously within another year or so of trying on their own. But we have not met many infertile couples willing to keep their lives perpetually on hold.

The procedure is usually scheduled based on the results of the urinary LH testing kit. Based on the woman's cycle, she is instructed when to begin testing and to schedule the insemination on the day following detection of the surge. The test is done in the afternoon or early evening so as not to miss the surge, which usually begins early in the day but may not be detectable in the urine until several hours later. One the day of insemination, the husband masturbates a specimen into a sterile, nontoxic plastic container. Preferably, the couple has avoided intercourse for two to three days before the anticipated day of insemination. After the specimen liquefies, it is washed in a nutrient medium. This can be done by a variety of techniques and in any one of several media. The washing procedure produces a concentrated pellet of motile sperm that is mixed with medium and placed into the uterus through the cervix by means of a thin plastic tube.

The wash and insemination are relatively inexpensive, currently costing around $100 per cycle. Side effects are rare but may include cramping. The risk of complications is low and related chiefly to the possibility of introducing infection. In fact, many physicians administer a prophylactic antibiotic at the time of the procedure to prevent infection.

Uterine Problems

While uterine problems are relatively uncommon causes of inability to conceive, they can cause miscarriage. Fibroids, if they are constricting the cavity and thought to be related to infertility or early pregnancy loss, can be removed. If they are on a stalk, removal by hysteroscopy is possible. This involves placing a telescope through the cervix under general anesthesia. Surgical instruments placed through channels in the scope can both cauterize and cut to remove certain types of fibroids. Hysteroscopy can also be used to cut adhesions bridging the uterine cavity (Asherman's syndrome) and to correct certain specific congenital abnormalities such as a uterine septum. Even though hysteroscopy is usually done as a day surgery, the costs are significant, totaling about $1500 to $2000.

If fibroids need to be removed through an abdominal incision, the procedure (abdominal myomectomy) would carry all the risks, recuperation time, and costs of any major abdominal surgery. Risks include bleeding, infection, and anesthesia. In addition, there would be the significant risk of the development of adhesions to the sites on the uterus where the fibroids were removed. Some surgeons are using a laser to make the incisions in the uterus to try to reduce inflammation around the incision, with hope of diminishing the tendency to form adhesions. Estimated costs of an abdominal myomectomy today would probably be in the area of $10,000, depending on medical costs in your area.

Endometrial infection with ureaplasma is treatable with the long-acting form of the antibiotic tetracycline (doxycycline). Both partners are treated for ten days with minimal cost and small chance of complications or side effects. Tuberculosis should be treated medically, but treatment will not result in resolution of the infertility and IVF will be required. The physical abnormalities caused by prenatal DES exposure currently cannot be treated directly, but other causes of infertility should be sought out. Treatments that increase the chance of a multiple pregnancy should be avoided as much as possible since DES-exposed individuals do not tolerate multiple pregnancy well.

Unexplained infertility

If none of the tests has shown an abnormality, the cause of the infertility is said to be unexplained. In some such couples there may be sperm defects or egg abnormalities that have not been detected by standard tests. For example, examination of sperm for more minor defects of sperm morphology (strict morphology) has shown that many failures of fertilization with IVF are explained by a very low percentage of sperm that are truly normal. In some cases this can be remedied in vitro by adding a large number of sperm to each egg. In other instances, the sperm may look normal but be unable to penetrate the egg. This possibility may be evaluated by testing the sperm with hamster eggs, but the importance of this factor can't be fully known until the sperm are placed with the woman's eggs. On the other side, we now know that some women have poor-quality eggs. However, in most couples with unexplained failure to conceive, it is a situation with normal sperm and eggs and the problem is that they are not meeting in adequate numbers to achieve fertilization.

The number of sperm getting to the egg and staying there may be decreased by either fewer coming up the genital tract or more being removed from around the egg by scavenger cells in the pelvis. Actually, the sperm don't make their way up the genital tract under their own steam, but require contractions of the woman's reproductive organs. Problems can be caused by alterations in the muscular movements of the uterus or lower-than-normal levels of contraction-producing substances in the man's semen. On the other hand, women with an infertility problem have increased numbers of scavenger cells (macrophages) in the pelvic cavity, which can reduce the numbers of sperm available. In other women the tubes may not have the normal capacity to pick up the egg. So, much unexplained infertility is now not really unexplained!

In line with these basic problems of getting sperm and eggs together, such patients are often advised to have a short course of IUI. Then, to increase the numbers of eggs available to meet the sperm, the ovaries are stimulated with hMG-HCG, as in the anovulatory patient. The use of hMG/IUI makes sense before going on to IVF because it yields over 30 percent success over three cycles at about half the cost of GIFT or IVF. Finally, GIFT or IVF is the most direct solution, wherein the eggs and sperm are placed directly together either in the fallopian tube or the laboratory.

Many well-meaning friends, family members, and even health professionals will give these couples advice to relax, forget it, or adopt a baby. Denise, thirty-eight, who recently had a baby girl after eight years of infertility, tubal surgery, and three IVF cycles, said, "If one more doctor told me to go on a vacation, I was going to scream."

Most of the time one of these conventional treatments will end up with the wife calling her husband with her positive pregnancy test in hand and exclaiming "Honey, it worked!" But when it doesn't, you get introduced to the alphabet soup of assisted reproduction.

seven

Alphabet Soup: Techniques

By the time you are ready to consider the techniques we call assisted reproduction, you may already have been through many years of evaluation and treatment. Now you are faced with a new veritable alphabet soup of choices. IVF? GIFT? ZIFT? PROST? TE(S)T? Which procedure should you choose?

In many cases, the selection of a procedure will be based on what type of problem is causing your infertility. But in some cases, especially when the cause of the infertility is unexplained or there is a male problem, several options may be available. The procedures which are clinically available currently include:

- IVF (In Vitro Fertilization). This is the most advanced procedure in the ART repertoire, where the egg and sperm are combined in the laboratory, incubated, and the resulting embryos are transferred into the woman's uterus. The acronym sometimes used for this procedure is IVF/ET or IVF/ER, indicating embryo transfer or replacement.
- GIFT (Gamete IntraFallopian Transfer). This procedure transfers a mixture of eggs and sperm into the fallopian tube, allowing fertilization to take place in the normal location.
- ZIFT (Zygote IntraFallopian Transfer). With this method fertilization takes place in vitro, but the resulting fertilized eggs (zygotes) are placed in the fallopian tube.
- PROST (PROnuclear Stage Tubal Transfer). A specific variation of

ZIFT, in this technique the embryo is in the pronuclear stage when it is transferred to the fallopian tube.
• TE(S)T (Tubal Embryo [Stage] Transfer). Another variation of ZIFT, in which an early divided embryo is transferred into the tube.

As you can see, many of these procedures are very similar and some procedures, as defined by certain groups, may overlap. In some cases both GIFT and IVF are done, with transfer of eggs and sperm into the tube, and embryos into the uterus. Alphabet soup indeed!

A GOOD DOSE OF REALITY

Before we embark on a thorough discussion of each of these techniques, a closer look at the chances of success and failure is in order. Remember, although the success rates of these procedures are improving, it is very important to have a realistic expectation of the chance of success. In fact, that's exactly what Dr. J. Benjamin Younger, president of the American Fertility Society (AFS), said in testimony before the House of Representatives Subcommittee on Regulation and Small Business Opportunities (which released the March 1989 survey of IVF/GIFT programs).

The congressional survey, which was developed in conjunction with the American Fertility Society and its affiliate Society for Assisted Reproductive Technology (SART), revealed that in 1987 the average IVF "take-home" baby rate was 11.6 percent per egg retrieval procedure and 13.3 percent per embryo transfer. The corresponding rate for GIFT was 15 percent per egg retrieval. The 1988 data from the Congressional survey suffered from some significant errors as we will point out later. Of course, the quoting of average figures obscures the most important finding in the survey—vast differences in success from one clinic to another, from a low of 0 percent to a high of 25 percent. During 1988, more than 16,000 IVF and/or GIFT procedures were performed in the United States by the 135 clinics reporting to the AFS registry. The "take home" baby rates were 12 and 21 percent for IVF and GIFT respectively per egg retrieval and 3,427 babies were born.

These statistics may not sound too encouraging on the surface. But, as indicated previously and as Dr. Younger pointed out before Congress, "a reproductively normal couple has [only] about a 20 percent chance of delivering a baby as a result of a single month's attempt and IVF patients are not reproductively normal." When you take that into account and add to that the fact that most of these couples were hopelessly infertile before this technology, those 1858 babies take on new meaning.

TECHNIQUES

IVF

The procedure of in vitro fertilization/embryo transfer consists of four basic steps:
1. Ripening of the egg(s)
2. Retrieval of the eggs
3. Fertilization of the eggs and growth of the resulting embryo(s)
4. Transfer of the embryo(s) into the uterus (ET)

Before a patient is placed into the program, certain tests should be done if they have not been done recently. We recommend a semen analysis, test for sperm antibodies in both husband and wife, sperm penetration assay, evaluation or treatment for chlamydia, and a "trial transfer." The transfer is the most critical part of the process and a rehearsal of this process with a mapping of the cervical canal is most useful.

Egg development

In the initial attempts at IVF, the natural cycle of the woman was used. After the first successes it became apparent that the efficiency of the process could be improved by the development of multiple eggs. Currently, there are a variety of stimulation regimens, including clomiphene with hMG/HCG (CC/hMG/HCG), hMG/HCG, and hMG/ HCG combined with a GnRH analog.

Until recently, CC/hMG/HCG was the most common regimen used. In most cases CC would be started on Day 2 or 3 of the cycle and continued for five days. The hMG was started before the CC was stopped (overlapping) or sometimes given simultaneously with the CC. A number of studies utilizing endometrial biopsy in women not going on to transfer have reported that the use of the CC interferes in some women with the development of secretory changes that prepare the endometrium for implantation of the embryo.

Somewhat less common has been the use of hMG/HCG without

CC. Again, stimulation is usually started on Day 2 or 3 of the cycle. The dose of hMG is higher, thus the number of daily injections and cost are also higher. Although no comparative study has been reported to prove greater success with avoiding the use of CC, we know that the retarded secretory development of the endometrium is prevented, and it has been empirically observed that some of the highest reported success rates have been by programs, including our own, using hMG without CC. In addition to hMG Metrodin (pure FSH) has also been utilized, with the theoretical advantage of lower LH levels during egg maturation.

With both of these regimens the main problem has been the response of the pituitary gland to the development of multiple follicles. Estrogen levels rise to concentrations higher than in a normal cycle, triggering the premature release of luteinizing hormone (LH). LH, in turn, may cause early aging of the eggs or even release of the eggs from the ovary. In those cycles with a full surge of LH, either the cycle must be canceled or egg retrieval must be timed by very frequent blood or urine LH measurements. In some cases there is a higher baseline level of LH without the surge, which has been associated with a lower rate of pregnancy.

A relatively new approach has been to suppress the pituitary with a GnRH agonist so that premature release of LH will not occur. This reduces the rate of cancellation in LH surge cycles, and the inconvenient frequent monitoring of LH is not necessary. A number of programs, including our own, have reported decreased cancellation rates along with increased pregnancy rates. Several recently published and some yet unpublished studies have show statistically significant increases of the pregnancy rate compared to CC/hMG/HCG and hMG/HCG without a GnRH agonist.

We have been using pretreatment with a GnRH agonist, leuprolide acetate (Lupron), combined with hMG/HCG for most of our ovarian stimulations for about three years. We feel that the use of Lupron provides more control over the stimulated cycle, an increased number of eggs and embryos, and probably better egg quality. Our rate of cancellation because of poor development of the follicles or a poor estrogen pattern has decreased from about 30 percent to about 10 percent. We feel that this latter advantage is the most important since the inconvenience and psychological impact of cycle cancellation is considerable. These factors, together with the cost of the canceled cycle, more than offset the increased drug costs with the combined treatment.

The cycle begins about a week following an ovulation that has been documented by a urinary ovulation-detector kit or a temperature chart. The patient comes in for an initial vaginal ultrasound scan to evaluate the baseline appearance of the pelvic organs and a urine test to prove that ovulation has occurred. If the scan is normal and the test shows evidence of ovulation, she is started on daily injections of Lupron subcutaneously (under the skin). These injections can be given by her husband or self-administered. After ten days of Lupron, or later if her menstrual period has not started, she returns for another scan and a blood test to see if her estrogen level is suppressed. A normal scan and suppressed estrogen level allow us to start her on hMG injections. The dose given is based on her weight or according to her previous individual response to hMG. Again, metrodin may be given instead of, or in combination with hMG. These injections are somewhat more difficult to give since they are a larger volume and are given deep in the muscle. It is rare that a person can self-administer this shot, so her husband or a friend is generally taught how to do this.

On the sixth day of hMG she returns for a scan, which may result in a modification of her dosage. Repeat scans are done every one to three days. When the follicles reach close to mature size, daily blood tests for estrogen and progesterone are done. When the size and number of the follicles and resulting estrogen level indicate that they are mature, HCG is given and preparations are made for retrieval of the eggs.

Egg retrieval

If the eggs are not retrieved within thirty-six hours of the HCG injection, spontaneous ovulation may occur. Therefore, the timing of the trigger injection of HCG is crucial. If we schedule the egg retrieval for 9:30 A.M. two days hence, instructions are given to take the HCG *precisely* at 11:00 P.M. The precise timing of this injection has led to a number of interesting situations.

One of our patients was a movie producer who had a preview of a major motion picture scheduled for the night his wife needed her HCG *precisely* at 9:00 P.M. They silently tiptoed out of the theater and looked for a place to give the injection. You may never have thought about this, but there are not many good places in a packed movie theater to give an injection. They ended up in the ladies' room, unpacked their syringe, needle, and vial of HCG. They mixed the HCG and she received her injection right on time. Both of them were hysterical when they realized that if anyone had happened to come into that room, she probably would have thought "Look at those Hollywood types. They can't even sit through a movie without shooting up!" Another similar situation occurred when a couple was required to attend a business meeting in a restaurant the night the HCG was given. Again, promptly at the assigned hour, the couple excused themselves, headed for a corner of the kitchen, and proceeded to "shoot up" to an amazed audience of waiters and busboys.

Nowadays, eggs are usually picked up by one of two methods. The earliest attempts were by laparoscopy, and some programs still do it that way. The trend, however, is definitely in the direction of ultrasound-directed retrieval. In 1985, laparoscopy was reported to account for 94.2 percent of egg retrievals. In 1986 it accounted for 78.2 percent and has decreased since that time; by 1988 only 13 percent were by laparoscopy, 86 percent by ultrasound, and the remainder by a combination of the two.

If the retrieval is by laparoscopy, an anesthesiologist will administer either a general or epidural anesthetic. The general anesthetic puts the patient to sleep with drugs and gas. The anesthesiologist must be careful not to use agents that may be toxic to the eggs. The epidural, which we prefer, is an injection of local anesthetic into a space near the spinal column. Little medication gets into the bloodstream, and toxicity is not a problem. The patient feels numb from the ribcage down and tolerates the laparoscopy well. The surgeon makes a small incision under the navel and inserts a telescope. Additional incisions are made to accommodate instruments to manipulate the ovaries and puncture the follicles to remove the eggs. Each follicle is punctured, the follicular fluid is removed, and then culture medium is flushed into the follicle and aspirated until the egg is found. The fluid is handed to an assistant, who passes it to the embryologist for screening. When the egg is identified, the next follicle is aspirated; this is continued until all the follicles have been emptied. When the procedure is finished, the incisions are closed with small stitches or paper strips.

Laparoscopy is considered an operative procedure. It requires an anesthetic and carries the risks of complications that can occur with any operation. That, however, is not to say it is an unsafe operation. But there is the chance of bleeding, infection, injury to the bowel or other organs, and reactions to the anesthetic. It also requires several days of recuperation. In order to make IVF a more economical and widespread technique, a search was begun for a more economical, safe, and acceptable procedure to retrieve the eggs.

The first attempts to achieve this were made by using abdominal ultrasound to guide a needle into the follicles of the ovary through the bladder, but this technique was technically difficult and painful. It was through the development of vaginal ultrasound probes that an alternative technique blossomed. The placement of the ultrasound probe into the vagina brought it very close to the ovary, thus giving a sharp image. The addition of the needle guide to the probe allowed fairly direct access to the ovaries. However, there are still some rare patients in whom the ovaries are inaccessible who need to have the retrieval done by laparoscopy. The advantages of ultrasound-guided follicle aspiration are that it is done with sedation rather than anesthesia and that it is not a full surgical procedure—with, consequently, less risk, expense, and recuperation time. Any of the complications mentioned with laparoscopy could occur with an ultrasound retrieval, but they would be less likely. You avoid the expense of an operating room, anesthesiologist, and assistant surgeon. Almost all patients who have experienced both methods of retrieval prefer the ultrasound route.

The patient is given Demerol and Valium preoperatively. An intravenous is started and the patient is positioned as she would be for a pelvic examination. The vagina and surrounding area are washed with an antiseptic solution. Paper drapes are then put around the area and the antiseptic is washed out of the vagina with culture fluid. (Many patients indicate that this preparation is the most uncomfortable part of the procedure.) The ultrasound probe is then covered with a sterile sheath, the needle guide is attached, and the probe is then placed in the vagina. The follicles are visualized on the screen. The needle is placed through the vaginal wall into the ovary and into the first follicle. The follicle is aspirated, flushed with medium, and reaspirated until the egg is found as in the laparosopic method. Each follicle is aspirated similarly. Once the needle is in the ovary, most patients do not feel any discomfort. In most patients, the preparation and the puncture of the vaginal wall cause the only significant pain in this procedure. After the procedure is completed, the patient is watched for a period of time before going home.

Most patients tolerate ultrasound retrieval very well. For someone very concerned about pain an epidural anesthetic is offered. But the majority of patients are awake and chatting during the procedure. We usually provide their favorite music by means of earphones to further relax them. During one memorable retrieval, the batteries in our tape player failed. The patient, an accomplished singer, entertained the staff with her repertoire of gospel music.

The number of eggs retrieved can vary tremendously. In March 1989 we reported an average of 11.7 eggs retrieved utilizing this stimulation protocol combined mostly with ultrasound retrieval. The harvest can vary up to 30 or more. You must remember, however, that this is not a numbers game. In general, the more eggs produced, the lower the average quality, although usually several good eggs are obtained. As the eggs are identified by the embryologist, they will be categorized according to apparent maturity and quality. What he or she is looking for are mature and good-quality eggs that will fertilize and form a good embryo. If many eggs are retrieved, many will be immature and will likely result in a poorer fertilization rate. It sounds great to say "I produced twenty-four eggs!" But remember that you are after a baby, not eggs. Don't be disappointed if there are only four which then fertilize. It's more important that those four are of good quality. Sometimes even one may be enough.

The night of the retrieval the patient is started on progesterone injections to prime the endometrium for implantation. Most patients who have been stimulated to form many eggs have estrogen levels far in excess of normal. The elevated level of estrogen needs to be balanced by higher amounts of progesterone to form an appropriate endometrium. The progesterone injections will be continued until fourteen days after embryo transfer, when the pregnancy test is done.

Fertilization

While the patient is being observed following the pick-up, the eggs are taken to the laboratory, where they are incubated until insemination. The incubation period allows some of the immature eggs to mature. At this time the embryologist may dissect some of the surrounding tissue away from the eggs if a previous problem with fertilization has occurred. The husband will produce a semen sample in a sterile container by masturbation. In some cases of male factor, an additional sample may be obtained one to two days before the retrieval. The specimen is washed, incubated, and then an appropriate number (usually 50,000 to 100,000) are placed in the medium with the egg.

Obtaining the semen specimen is a crucial part of the process. It would seem fairly straightforward for a man who probably has provided countless previous specimens for testing and insemination. But, as Murphy's Law states "Whatever can go wrong probably will." We know of a number of incidents in which an adequate specimen was not forthcoming. Rarely, a man simply may not be able to perform under the tremendous stress of the importance of this particular specimen. We have, on occasion, had the wife quickly recover from her retrieval to help her husband obtain the specimen. And there have been times when in the excitement of the moment the specimen missed the cup and landed on the floor.

Perhaps the most unusual incident involved a couple who were Orthodox Jews. According to their beliefs, masturbation is not permitted and all previous specimens had been collected by intercourse, using a nontoxic condom. That's not a problem. But it was also their belief that the husband could not have intercourse with his wife until a certain period of time after her menses and only after she participated in a ritual bath. In their first attempt at IVF, her follicles came along very quickly and the day of retrieval was scheduled before she would be allowed to take the ritual bath. After much soul-searching, the couple elected not to take the HCG and aborted the cycle. When problems are anticipated, we generally freeze a specimen, but unfortunately the sperm did not freeze well in this case. (At the April 1989 IVF World Congress in Jerusalem, one of Israel's leading rabbis addressed the meeting and indicated that it was his interpetation that exceptions could be made to those types of rules if a greater good is to be achieved through the procedure.)

Assuming that sperm can be obtained and the eggs inseminated, the next morning the eggs will be examined for evidence of fertilization. We hope to see two structures in each egg, the male and female pronuclei, indicating that fertilization has taken place. At this time abnormal eggs, those which may have fertilized with more than one sperm, will be discarded. Those which did not fertilize will be inseminated again and fertilization will be checked the next day.

One day later—two days after the retrieval—the eggs are checked again. This time we are looking for evidence that the fertilized eggs, now embryos, have divided. They will be scored according to their number of cells and other characteristics. The previously unfertilized eggs will be checked again for evidence of fertilization. Selection will be made on the basis of embryo morphology (appearance) as to which will be:

- Discarded because they did not fertilize or are abnormal
- Frozen for future use if the couple chose this option (actually we now freeze most at the pronuclear stage)
- Transferred into the uterus

The selection of how many embryos to transfer and which ones to use takes a great deal of experience. Most couples elect to have three or four embryos transferred into the uterus. This number is a good balance between success and avoidance of multiple pregnancy. Curiously, the rate of multiple pregnancy has been higher than one would calculate it should be. This led to the suggestion that additional embryos actually help each other develop, implant, and thereby increase the chance of success. The chance of multiple pregnancy increases in proportion to the success rate of a program, as it is an index of embryo quality and therefore the quality of the laboratory. Circumstances leading to a reduced number of embryos being transferred might include:

- A small uterine cavity that cannot carry a multiple pregnancy well
- Age below 35, which makes more than one embryo implanting likely
- Excellent-quality embryos

The selection of the particular embryos to be transferred is based on experience. The physical characteristics considered favorable are:

- Greater number of cells
- Uniform size and shape of the cells
- Absence of fragmentation of the cells
- Areas of thinning of the zona (shell)

But, in the final analysis, these factors only lead to tendencies toward a better implantation. We know that sometimes very irregular embryos can develop into healthy pregnancies. So, although we can try to limit the risk of multiple pregnancy, currently we simply do not have the means to tell which embryos will implant.

Which should be transferred and which frozen? Our philosophy is to transfer the best embryos, since it is far better, practically and psychologically, to conceive during the IVF cycle. Some programs freeze the best embryos, but we do not feel there is any current proof that an embryo will do better by being replaced later.

Embryo transfer (replacement)

About forty-eight hours after these microscopic eggs were retrieved through a needle they are transferred back into the woman's body. But now, they are embryos with all the genetic material they need to develop from their current two- to eight-cell size into an adult human being.

The woman is given Valium orally about an hour before the transfer. She is placed in the pelvic examination position in a darkened, quiet room. Her mate sits by her side, holding her hand. The incubator holding the embryos to be transferred is quietly wheeled into the room. As a speculum is placed in the vagina, the husband has an opportunity to come over to the incubator to look through the microscope and view his offspring. This is a special moment, a very emotional one for the husband. After all those years, tests, treatments, and disappointments, there they are—three or four embryos, any or all of which have the potential to develop into their children. After the husband rejoins his wife the embryos are drawn up into a small plastic catheter that has been bent into a proper shape to enter the uterus through the cervix. The cervix is washed by the doctor and the catheter is placed according to a map drawn during a trial transfer done prior to this cycle. The embryos are expelled from the catheter. The catheter is withdrawn and the patient rests in the transfer bed for about three hours. In fact, she is instructed to stay in bed for the next two days and then avoid strenuous activity, exercise, and intercourse for the next two weeks until the pregnancy test.

Success and failure

Not every patient who enters the program completes the cycle. Cancellation of the cycle can occur during any of the four stages. We have cited several instances above. However, most cancellations will occur during the stimulation. These may be the result of:

- Development of only one follicle
- Failure of any follicles to develop
- Development of too many small follicles, resulting in a very high estrogen level that will tend to inhibit implantation and possibly lead to overstimulation

At times, poor fertilization may result in not having any embryos to transfer. We recently had a patient who had gone through several unsuccessful cycles elsewhere who developed six follicles. Six eggs were retrieved but only three fertilized. On the second day it was noted that none of the fertilized eggs had divided, which is extremely unusual. One of the previously unfertilized eggs had fertilized. The transfer was postponed until the next day, when only the egg that had fertilized on the second try had divided. From six promising eggs, only one embryo was available for transfer. That lone embryo was transferred on the third day following retrieval, but with only a very small chance of success. The odds against that lone embryo were too high. She did not get pregnant. In her case it was now obvious that her multiple failed cycles involved poor-quality eggs, whereas their previous poor performance had been attributed only to a sperm problem. The appearance of her eggs to the experienced eye was very unusual, and microscopic studies are now being done. She was matched with an egg donor. As you will see in Chapter 11, she will now have an excellent chance of success.

Assuming a couple completes the cycle, what are their chances of pregnancy? According to the 1988 annual report of the U.S. Registry of IVF-ET with 135 centers reporting, the clinical pregnancy rate was sixteen percent and "take-home" baby rate was 12 percent per retrieval. The same data resulted in a 19 percent clinical pregnancy rate and a 14 percent "take-home" baby rate per transfer. Five percent of all pregnancies were ectopic. Multiple deliveries occured in 19 percent of the clinical pregnancies, with 2.9 percent resulting in triplets or more. (For the success rates of individual programs as reported to the congressional survey, see Appendix 1.)

"NATURAL CYCLE" IVF

The first attempts and success with IVF were performed within the woman's natural cycle. In an attempt to make the process more efficient the various stimulation protocols were developed. Now many reproductive specialists believe that there is a legitimate place in today's practice of assisted reproduction for "natural cycle" IVF. Its benefits include lower costs, fewer injections, better acceptability for women who may have ethical or religious problems with embryo freezing and the disposition of extra embryos, and virtually no risk of multiple pregnancy. With the lower cost a couple can go through more cycles.

Egg development

From a technical standpoint, the major difference between stimulated and natural cycles would be that more intensive monitoring of the natural cycle is substituted for the monitoring and stimulation with fertility drugs. No Lupron or Pergonal is given. Vaginal ultrasound examinations are begun on a day calculated according to the woman's shortest menstrual interval. Once the dominant follicle reaches close to mature size, her blood will be measured daily for estradiol and LH levels. Urine specimens obtained at frequent intervals will be checked for evidence of the LH surge. When the follicle reaches mature size before the surge is detected, an HCG injection will be given and the retrieval will be scheduled for thirty-five hours later (Figure 13). If the surge is detected before the HCG is given, the HCG will be given and the retrieval scheduled based on the estimated time of the surge.

Retrieval

The retrieval will be performed with the use of the vaginal ultrasound probe just as in stimulated cycles. But the fact that only one follicle is being retrieved means that less sedation is necessary, an IV is not started, and the observation period after the procedure is shorter.

Fertilization

Fertilization technique is identical to that in stimulated cycles but, of course, only one egg is available for insemination.

Transfer

Transfer technique is identical to stimulated cycles, but with the advantage that the endometrium is more favorable for implantation since it is not overstimulated by the estrogen produced by multiple follicles.

Success and failure

Recently it has been shown by two European groups that retrieval of one mature egg in a normal menstrual cycle has been associated with a clinical pregnancy rate of about 20 percent. It remains to be seen whether these favorable results can be duplicated.

GIFT

GIFT stands for Gamete IntraFallopian Transfer. The sperm and eggs (gametes) are placed together and transferred into the fallopian tube by means of a catheter during a laparoscopy. The apparent differences between IVF and GIFT are that GIFT requires that the tubes be open. Obstructed fallopian tubes are one of the primary reasons for performing IVF. In GIFT, fertilization takes place in its normal location, the fallopian tube. It also eliminates the most difficult part of IVF, the embryo transfer. GIFT has resulted in better overall pregnancy rates and therefore has enjoyed increasing popularity.

As of July 1988 the procedure was no longer viewed as an experimental procedure, according to the American Fertility Society (AFS). The AFS felt that GIFT could be considered a standard clinical procedure if:

- The patient and her partner have been investigated using AFS minimum standards.
- The patient has at least one normal fallopian tube and a condition not amenable to less invasive techniques.
- The facility performing the procedure has a laboratory and personnel that meet the AFS's minimum standards for IVF.
- GIFT is performed in a facility that is prepared to carry out IVF as an alternative if GIFT does not prove a feasible option.

These are good rules to remember and to apply to a program if you are considering GIFT.

Basically, a GIFT cycle consists of three steps:
- Development and ripening of the eggs
- Retrieval of the eggs
- Transfer of the eggs and washed sperm into the fallopian tube

Before a patient enters a GIFT program, the same basic tests may be done as those carried out prior to an IVF cycle. The only exception is that there is no absolute need to perform a trial transfer, since an embryo transfer would not be anticipated unless the fallopian tubes were found to be closed. Documentation that the tubes are open may be prudent if that fact has not been confirmed recently. The main reasons for performing GIFT are prolonged infertility as the result of:

• Unexplained infertility
• Endometriosis
• The male factor

Egg Development

In order to achieve maximal efficiency of the GIFT process, stimulation of the ovaries similar to that for IVF will usually be carried out in order that an average of four eggs can be transferred to the fallopian tube. As in IVF, stimulation protocols can vary considerably among programs. But, in general, the administration of the drugs and monitoring of the cycles with ultrasound and estrogen levels are similar to what we described with IVF.

Egg retrieval

Once the HCG is given, the retrieval is scheduled thirty-four to thirty-five hours later. It is done by laparoscopy since this is the means by which the eggs will be replaced in the tube. (Refer back to page 102 for the details of this procedure.)

Transfer

The difference between this and the laparoscopy for IVF is that after the eggs are retrieved, the embryologist will categorize them as to quality and maturity, select the best for transfer, and load them together with sperm into a special catheter for placement into the tube. The catheter will then be passed through one of the instruments and carefully placed into the fallopian tube. Usually three to four eggs and appropriate numbers of sperm are then injected through the catheter into the fallopian tube, allowing fertilization to occur in its normal place in the body. The embryos then make their own way down the tube and into the uterus for implantation.

When the procedure was first developed and until recently, half the eggs and sperm were placed in each fallopian tube. That is, if four eggs were transferred, two with appropriate numbers of sperm would be placed in each tube. Recently, higher pregnancy rates have been reported by transferring all the eggs and sperm into one of the tubes.

Success and Failure

The average chance of a GIFT procedure resulting in a live birth is greater than that for IVF, although not all patients treatable by IVF are candidates for GIFT. The most significant problem that cannot be treated with GIFT is, of course, tubal obstruction. In 1988, the U.S. Registry reported the clinical pregnancy rate was 27 percent; the delivery rate was 21 percent. The multiple pregnancy rate was 30 percent with 5.8 percent being more than twins. Of the total pregnancies, 5 percent were ectopic. The spontaneous miscarriage rate for GIFT was 20 percent.

There is, according to this report, a great variation in success and in clinics doing GIFT, five clinics accounted for 37 percent of the deliveries. The implications for the consumer are obvious. For programs with a good IVF laboratory and physicians experienced with operative laparoscopy, achieving good success with GIFT is not difficult, but neither of these prerequisites can be assumed.

ZIFT, PROST, AND TE(S)T

These three procedures are similar in that they are all variations of basic GIFT, except that instead of sperm and eggs, fertilized eggs (zygotes) of various stages are placed in the fallopian tube. The advantage is to allow the embryos to spend time in the natural environment of the fallopian tube and then enter the uterus in the normal manner, without the potential adverse effects of the embryo transfer. The benefit of placing embryos rather than sperm and eggs is that you then know that fertilization has occurred and you avoid one drawback of the GIFT procedure. Also, fertilization occurs more reliably in the laboratory, where a high concentration of sperm can be placed close to the egg. This is especially useful if the problem is a male factor or if you have unexplained infertility, both of which have a reduced chance of fertilization.

ZIFT will consist of four parts:
• Development and ripening of the eggs
• Retrieval of the eggs
• Fertilization of the egg and growth of the embryo
• Placement of the embryo into the fallopian tube

Egg Development

The stimulation protocol for these procedures will vary, depending upon the preferences of a particular program. Basically, the same drugs and monitoring will be employed as for IVF or GIFT.

Egg retrieval

The use of transvaginal ultrasound-directed retrieval has allowed for the development of these procedures, since it is fairly simple and tolerated well under local anesthesia and/or sedation.

Fertilization

Again, the eggs and sperm would be brought together in the laboratory and fertilization would be "in vitro" as in IVF.

Placement in the tube

This is the aspect in which these procedures differ from IVF. Depending upon which stage of embryo is going to be selected for placement in the fallopian tube, a laparoscopy would be scheduled at the proper interval from the retrieval. For example, in PROST (Pronuclear Stage Transfer), the embryologist will examine the eggs in fifteen to twenty hours for evidence of the formation of two pronuclei, which is a sign that fertilization has taken place. These pronuclear embryos are then placed in the fallopian tube by the same technique as in GIFT. Under laparoscopic guidance, a catheter is passed into the end of the tube and the embryos gently expelled. When dividing embryos are placed in the tube, the term TE(S)T (Tubal Embryo Stage Transfer) has been used.

Success and Failure

The 1988 registry results were the first to include ZIFT. Of the 355 egg retrieval cycles, 27 percent resulted in clinical pregnancy, and 20 percent in delivery, 32 percent of them multiple. These results were virtually identical to those of GIFT, indicating that the advantage of ZIFT is mainly in assuring and documenting fertilization in cases where the chance of fertilization is in doubt.

Frozen Embryos (Cryopreservation)

One of the developments in assisted reproduction that has the potential to significantly increase the efficiency of IVF procedures is embryo freezing (cryopreservation). Sperm freezing has been routine for some time and techniques to freeze embryos are currently being employed in many programs. In the future, procedures may be developed for practical freezing of eggs.

Since we now have the technology to stimulate the production of many eggs and have efficient techniques to retrieve those eggs and fertilize them, the ability to freeze the embryos and utilize them in multiple cycles should greatly improve efficiency. One stimulation and retrieval can provide embryos not only for a transfer during that IVF cycle but also for additional frozen embryo transfer cycles.

A perfect example of this ability is the story of Jane and Terry Mohr. The story of the birth of their "triplets" twenty-one months apart was reported nationwide and described in detail in *Redbook* magazine. Jane's first pregnancy at age thirty-three was an ectopic pregnancy in the left tube. Her second pregnancy was discovered to be ectopic, this time in the right fallopian tube. The tube was surgically opened, the pregnancy removed, and the tube was repaired. Her third pregnancy, stimulated by clomiphene, was also ectopic, in the right tube. By this time, after three ectopic pregnancies, her doctor referred her for in vitro fertilization, fearing that her tubes were too severely damaged to try again.

She entered the UCLA IVF program and on June 26, 1986, ten eggs were retrieved. Nine of those eggs fertilized and four were implanted into her uterus two days following the retrieval. The remaining five were frozen. On February 15, 1987, their son Cooper, weighing 3 pounds 14 ounces, was born by caesarean section in her eighth month of pregnancy when she developed toxemia. When Dr. Meldrum moved his program to Redondo Beach, the Mohrs asked that their frozen embryos also be moved, since they lived close to the new center. In March 1988, Jane returned to have her frozen embryos transferred. Three of the five had survived the freeze and thaw and were transferred into the uterus. On November 29, 1988, twin daughters, Hannah Christina and Mollie McKenna, both weighing more than 5 pounds, were born. Cooper and the twin girls are technically triplets, conceived during the same cycle but, through assisted reproductive technology, born almost two years apart. More recently we have had two further "twins," the second being born forty months after the first retrieval.

Freezing of embryos is an option all couples going through IVF should consider. Even by those who have no ethical problems with embryo freezing many decisions have to be made regarding disposition of the frozen embryos in the event of divorce or death—or even a cross-country move. In divorce the couple may choose to assign the embryos to one or another of them, donate them to another couple, or discard them. In case of death of one, the other member of the couple could take possession. At the death of both, the frozen embryos could be donated or discarded. Difficult as this is to think about, these decisions must be made prior to the actual procedure.

The most unusual situation regarding frozen embryos was the widely publicized case of Risa and Steven York. In 1986, the Yorks went through an IVF program at the Jones Institute for Reproductive Medicine in Norfolk, Virginia. After failed attempts at IVF and frozen embryo transfers, the Yorks moved from New Jersey to California and requested that their one remaining frozen embryo be transferred to a comparable facility in Los Angeles. The Jones Institute refused and offered them four choices. They could have the embryo transferred at the Jones Institute or have it donated to another couple, destroyed, or used for experimentation.

The Yorks sued, but a federal judge refused to grant a preliminary injunction and ordered a trial to begin some time later. This is a problem for Mrs. York, thirty-nine, since increasing age may reduce her chance of becoming pregnant. This case raises the question "Just whose embryo is it?" The mother's, the father's, or the doctor's? We believe that a couple's embryos are the property of the couple and decisions as to the disposition must remain their sole right. But, happily for the Yorks, this matter did not go to court. A settlement was reached in September 1989 whereby the clinic released the embryo and the Yorks released the clinic from any liability and agreed to drop their $200,000 lawsuit for emotional stress.

The nation's population of frozen embryos is now more than 4000 and growing. There are bound to be other conflicts like that between Mary Sue and Junior Davis. In this divorce case, Mary Sue wants to keep the embryos in storage in case she wants to use them or donate them to another couple. Junior Davis wants them destroyed because he feels that their use after the divorce would force him into unwanted fatherhood. If that happens, would he have to pay child support? Logically, the embryos would be treated as property in a divorce settlement, to be awarded to the partner with the predominating cause of fertility. However, at the trial court level the case was decided in favor of Mary Sue, based on the judge's ruling that the embryos were children and custody was awarded based on child custody law. The case is now on appeal.

Most of the time there is no conflict. The couple usually has a single purpose—to have a baby and frozen embryos can increase their chances. The frozen embryo transfer consists of four steps:

- Freezing of the embryos not being transferred during the IVF cycle
- Storage of the embryos
- Monitoring of the frozen embryo cycle
- Thawing of the embryos and transfer to the uterus

Freezing

Various programs differ on which embryos to freeze. Some freeze the best; others transfer the best embryos fresh during the IVF cycle. The rationale for freezing the best embryos is that in the IVF cycle the estrogen levels are very high and this somewhat interferes with the implantation process. Also, the best embryos will be more likely to survive the freezing process. Thus these groups reason that you should save the best embryos for a natural cycle when the hormones are nearest to normal. That seems to make sense. But it would seem better for the couple to conceive during the actual IVF cycle rather than to fail and require further treatment. Thus the vast majority of groups feel that they want to utilize the best embryos within the IVF cycle to give the patient the best chance of pregnancy in that cycle. This also seems to make sense. What some groups are now doing is a middle ground. When there are enough fertilized eggs at the pronuclear stage, they freeze some at this favorable time. But before cell division, the better embryos can't be consistently identified, so some of the better ones end up being frozen.

There may be some specific instances when the stimulated endometrium or the quality of the luteal phase may prevent implantation in the IVF cycle itself. Take for instance a recent couple in our program who experienced two very early (biochemical pregnancy) losses. Her embryo quality was good and we speculated that difficulty with implantation might be the problem. In her third cycle we emphasized freezing. She is now carrying twins from these frozen embryos transferred in a natural cycle. In her specific case, she produced very high-quality embryos, but her stimulated endometrium was the problem.

Storage

The embryos are maintained in a frozen state in liquid nitrogen with an alarm to prevent inadvertent thawing due to, for example, rare failure of the insulation of the storage tank. The embryos can be maintained in a frozen state indefinitely, but the longest frozen with successful implantation is so far forty months, again in a patient Dr. Meldrum first treated at UCLA and then later at his new facility. Provided they are kept immersed, they will probably remain unchanged for the reproductive life of the woman, which is the current ethical guideline in the United States for the duration of storage.

Monitoring the frozen embryo cycle

As you would expect, we do not want to place these valuable embryos into the uterus unless the endometrium is perfectly primed for implantation with the correct hormonal sequence of a normal ovulatory cycle. So the cycle is monitored with ultrasound to document the development of the follicle as well as with measurements of LH. The time of ovulation then can be precisely determined and the timing of the thawing of the embryos and their placement into the uterus planned. If the patient is not ovulating normally, a stimulated cycle, or a programmed cycle with the administration of appropriate hormones, may be necessary.

Thawing and transfer

Once ovulation has been determined or progesterone has been begun, the thaw of the embryos is scheduled. The timing of the thaw and transfer is based on the age of the embryos. Currently, about 50 percent of the embryos survive the freeze and thaw. In general, the more extra embryos available, the lower the percentage. Enough viable embryos are thawed until there are an adequate number (up to four) for the transfer. Of course, multiple pregnancy could be completely eliminated by transfer of one embryo each cycle, but this is less practical, particularly for couples coming from a distance. The transfer procedure is carried out in the same manner as in the IVF cycle we previously described.

Success and failure

In 1988, the success rate for frozen embryo transfer cycles was a 10 percent clinical pregnancy rate and a 7 percent "take-home" baby rate. But remember that these patients did not have to go through stimulation or retrieval. Instead of looking at this rate only, we should actually add this 7 percent to the success rates of the IVF cycles from which they resulted. (Keep in mind that only about half of couples have extra embryos to freeze.) Again, the programs doing more procedures had better success, with four groups which performed over fifty frozen cycles accounting for 49 percent of the deliveries by this method for a delivery rate of 15 percent compared to an average of 7 percent.

IVF OR GIFT: WHICH TO CHOOSE?

GIFT and the other procedures which utilize the fallopian tube for supporting gametes and embryos arose out of the frustration with low rates of success with IVF. Unless the IVF laboratory is functioning at a very high level, the fallopian tube is actually a better environment for the nourishment and growth of these cells. It is clearly evident, for example, that the transfer of eggs and sperm to the tube is more successful than IVF for the average U.S. program, since the rate of ongoing pregnancy with GIFT exceeded that with IVF by about 7 percent in 1986, 3 percent in 1987, and 9 percent in 1988. However, many programs' individual rates for IVF approached or exceeded the national average for GIFT, suggesting that high quality IVF approaches the results with GIFT. The comparison is further complicated by the fact that different groups of patients are appropriate for the two procedures. In one study the same group of patients was allocated to either IVF or GIFT and the success rates were identical.

At first glance, the GIFT procedure seems inherently more logical. First, it would seem that fertilization and embryo development must occur more normally in the location where these events usually take place. Second, the embryos do not reach the uterine cavity prematurely in GIFT, whereas in IVF, embryos have been routinely transferred to the uterus after about forty-eight hours to avoid prolonged exposure to potentially suboptimal culture conditions. Third, the embryos enter the uterus in a normal manner, without irritation and potential displacement of the embryos from the upper part of the uterus where implantation normally occurs.

However, these benefits are counterbalanced by inherent advantages of IVF. First, from animal studies, it appears that a lower percentage of eggs become normally fertilized with GIFT than with IVF. Since the eggs are aspirated from the ovary several hours before they would normally ovulate, these less-than-fully mature eggs may not fertilize or may fertilize abnormally. You would not know this with GIFT since you can't observe fertilization. Also, a much lower concentration of sperm is achieved in direct contact with the egg than in IVF, due to a very large area within the folds of the tube. Second, if pregnancy does not occur and extra eggs do not fertilize, there is no way to know whether the failure was due to lack of fertilization or of implantation. It is possible that in a good IVF program these factors balance off the advantages of GIFT and result in similar rates of success.

The other major difference between IVF and GIFT is the need for laparoscopy for the latter as well as a major form of anesthesia. For most women who have had prior surgeries and anesthesia, the prospect of a procedure without incisions and under local anesthesia is enough to offset a small increase of pregnancy with GIFT. On the other hand, laparoscopy adds significant diagnostic aspects and the possibility of treatment for some women. Endometriosis may be evaluated and cauterized or vaporized and the status of the tubes and adhesions can be assessed. In the recent case of one GIFT procedure we cauterized endometriosis and washed the pelvic cavity to remove the sperm-engulfing scavenger cells (macrophages) that are thought to reduce infertility in this disease. Although pregnancy did not occur with the GIFT, she conceived on her own the following month, after seven years of infertility and multiple cycles of hMG/IUI.

One further difference between IVF and GIFT is the risk of tubal pregnancy. Although surveys have shown virtually equal rates (about 5 percent of pregnancies), tubal pregnancies with IVF occur almost exclusively in women with abnormal tubes, whereas most women undergoing GIFT have normal tubes. Therefore, in the women for whom either GIFT or IVF is appropriate there is probably a small increase in the risk of ectopic pregnancy with GIFT. In women with tubal disease, the risk of ectopic pregnancy with GIFT varies from 5 percent to 17 percent, depending upon the extent of the tubal damage.

You can see that the choice of GIFT versus IVF is not easy and depends upon the success rate achieved with IVF in a particular program, the potential for diagnostic information, and the patient's outlook toward surgery, anesthesia, and tubal pregnancy.

Then what about ZIFT/PROST/TE(S)T? It is not clear whether

ZIFT/ PROST/ TE(S)T carries a higher rate of pregnancy than GIFT. It may be considered an option when a male factor or the presence of antisperm antibodies could impair fertilization with GIFT. Fertilization is more certain, as with IVF, and the placement of embryos into the tubes allows a further one to two days of development in the normal location and a normal entry into the uterus. However, it requires *both* transvaginal egg retrieval and laparoscopy, with accompanying increased discomfort and expense. The increased pregnancy rate is likely to be proportional to the increased cost, but a patient might rather save those financial resources for a further IVF cycle and avoid the increased discomfort of an operative procedure.

If your tubes are blocked, the choice is easy. IVF is the only appropriate method for you. If your problem is unrelated to a tubal factor, you have a choice. Now, you also have the facts. To summarize:

	IVF	GIFT	ZIFT	PROST	TET
Laparoscopy mandatory	—	+	+	+	+
Anesthesia mandatory	—	+	+	+	+
Ultrasound retrieval	+	—	+	+	+
Fertilization known	+	—	+	+	+
Fertilization in normal location	—	+	—	—	—
Requires normal fallopian tube	—	+	+	+	+
Diagnostic information	—	+	+	+	+

COSTS

An article in the March 1989 issue of *Changing Times* ("The High Cost of Fighting Infertility") estimated the cost of an IVF cycle at $4000 to $6000. Actually, with a recent price increase in the cost of hMG, the actual cost is probably now greater. What hurts most is that, unlike many other high-tech medical procedures, insurance usually does not pay for IVF. Some insurance companies specifically exclude IVF or may try to argue that IVF is elective or not medically necessary or not treating the underlying problem. A 1987 survey by the Health Insurance Association of America of its member companies found that 25 percent of them covered IVF under group policies. Of those companies that did cover it, only 25 percent did so as a standard practice. The rest review each claim individually.

Only six states mandate some coverage for infertility services at this time. If you live in Arkansas, California, Hawaii, Massachusetts, Maryland, or Texas you are lucky enough to be covered for some services. Only Massachusetts currently requires that IVF and other infertility treatments not considered experimental be covered to the same degree that other pregnancy-related procedures are. However, in Massachusetts GIFT is considered experimental and IVF is not. In Maryland, IVF is covered, but artificial insemination is not. Hawaii allows only one IVF cycle and Arkansas sets a lifetime cap of $15,000 on infertility treatments. The insurance situation is changing rapidly in many states as infertility support groups, physicians, and other interested parties lobby their state legislatures to have basic infertility and assisted reproductive procedures mandated in health insurance coverage. Court decisions in some states have held that these procedures must be covered if not specifically excluded. Of course, many insurance companies have already rewritten their contracts to exclude these services. In one notable case, the Kaiser Health Plan in California was forced by a class action suit to provide IVF for those years that it was a clinically accepted therapy but not specifically excluded in their contract.

Even if you are not eligible for infertility services, many tests and procedures can be indirectly covered as they legitimately relate to the treatment of disease. For example, if a laparoscopy that is being done to evaluate infertility uncovers and treats endometriosis or tubal disease, you might want to apply for benefits based on the disease found. Legal advice might be useful in determining your rights under your health insurance contract.

As of this writing, you can expect to spend from $4000 to $8000 for one of the ART procedures. There is great geographic variation in the costs, as well as some differences among programs in different parts of the same city. ZIFT/PROST/TE(S)T will be more expensive because they require independent expensive procedures for both egg retrieval and transfer. The cost of freezing and maintaining embryos is relatively small as opposed to going through another complete cycle to get more embryos. It is usually about $1000 for the freezing, storage fee, and the frozen embryo transfer cycle.

Our "take-home" message regarding costs is to ask for a full accounting of what your charges will be and when you will be expected to pay them. Most programs will have you pay up front because of the high costs of running an ART program and the uncertainty and delay of insurance payments.

Now that you are knowledgeable about the procedures and their costs, on what basis should you choose a physician, group, or IVF or GIFT program that most closely meets your needs? The next chapter tells you.

eight

Dr. Perfect, I Presume?

Y ou need the full arsenal of the informed, clear-headed consumer when you set out on your quest for the practitioner and program best equipped to help you do battle with infertility. Basic armament includes your knowledge that not all doctors are equally competent and that you need the services and understanding of one who is professionally excellent. You also know that cooperation and patience are going to be required on your part and you should realize that once in a while the wrong chemistry between medical expert and client couple can sabotage an otherwise promising therapeutic plan. And you admit, however sadly, that *the* Dr. Perfect practices only on Fantasy Island.

Your first determination has to be the type of doctor or program you need. This will depend to a great extent where you are in the process of investigating your infertility problem. If you have never consulted a physician for your problem or have not had many tests, your own gynecologist is probably the best place to begin. He or she will probably be board-certified or a candidate for certification by the American Board of Obstetrics and Gynecology and may be a member of a national fertility society such as the American Fertility Society. Membership in these organizations does not in itself mean that he or she is a great doctor but it does signify certain levels of training, experience, and interest in treating problems like yours. So read those diplomas while waiting to see the doctor and ask if they are not displayed. If you do not have your own gynecologist, read on. Most of the selection criteria and investigation we suggest will pertain to physicians with any level of specialization.

If you have already been through the basic testing and have tried various treatments, it may be time to move on. Now you may want to seek a more specialized level of care from a physician who has had special training in reproductive medicine. He or she will be certified or a candidate for certification by the American board in the specialized area of reproductive endocrinology. This means that he or she has spent at least two extra years in a fellowship devoted exclusively to study in this field and usually limits his or her practice to this specialty. These specialists can be found in individual practice, medical groups, fertility centers, and as directors of IVF programs.

SOURCES OF REFERRAL

You may or may not be under the care of a physician when you initiate your search for your own fertility specialist. You may be locked into a provider network through an HMO or PPO-type insurance, which will significantly limit or eliminate the possibility of making a choice. You may be in a geographic area that has half a dozen IVF centers, or you may live in a rural area where a great deal of travel is required to reach any center. The following are referral sources generally available, some less effective than others:

• YELLOW PAGES—In general, we do not suggest that you let your fingers do the walking to find any type of sophisticated medical service, especially ART. In fact, it's probably not a good idea to use the classified yellow pages to select any sort of health provider since you cannot obtain objective information from an advertisement. Certainly, the size of the ad is not in any way proportional to the quality of service or medical care you will receive. The yellow pages or ads in newspapers and magazines are probably okay to use in finding names and addresses of potential providers available. But remember that this may be an incomplete list; some of the best providers may choose not to advertise.

• MEDICAL ASSOCIATIONS—One method of selection often used is the physician referral service of the county medical association. We don't think this one is very good either. It is true that you will obtain the names of providers who are licensed and in "good standing" in the medical association. This means that they have paid their dues to the association and have not done a deed dastardly enough to get them thrown out, but it is no guarantee of quality. In addition, someone who comes very close to being your Dr. Perfect may choose not to be a member of this organization. The local medical association may be helpful to check out if any complaints have been filed against a particular physician, but it is not a good basis for making a selection.

- **PHYSICIAN REFERRAL SERVICE**—The same caveat is probably valid for physician referral services run by hospitals. These are purely mechanisms for bringing patients into that particular hospital's orbit. The referral service of a quality hospital is a step up from the medical association because the hospital, at least, has certain requirements for staff membership in the areas of education and training and requires references and monitoring for new physicians, so a certain minimum level of quality is assured. But, you're not looking for minimum standards. You're looking for excellence. Also, the referral service usually gives you the next three names on the list rather than one who meets your individual needs. Lately, some hospitals have been trying to meet more individual needs by using computer programs to match doctor and patient. The criteria used range from age of physician to schools attended and geographic location. This is somewhat helpful, but don't stop here.
- **FRIEND**—Asking a friend for a recommendation is actually a pretty good way to start the selection process and is light years better than a referral from the county medical association. This is because at least some objective criteria can be used. But you have to dig further and establish the reasons for the referral. The friend's referral is based more on his or her needs than yours. Start making your list of what you want in a doctor or program and make sure that your friend is making the referral based on what you think is important. Chances are you'll find a competent physician as well as one who is personable.
- **SUPPORT GROUPS**—Since the development of Alcoholics Anonymous, support groups have helped individuals and families with diverse medical problems. Infertility is no exception. The most prominent support group for couples with infertility is RESOLVE, Inc., headquartered

in Massachusetts. They provide education, support groups, a bi-
monthly newsletter, library and referral service, and have a nationwide network of chapters in most major cities. They are some of the
best-informed people about the infertility situation in your area.

• **YOUR PHYSICIAN**—If you are currently under the care of a physician
and he or she has offered you all the skill and expertise available to
him or her, the next step would be to refer you to a higher-level
expert to continue your care. This is a pretty good way to find a
physician but it does not mean that you can close your eyes and
blindly charge off to the new Dr. Right. Your doctor could have
referred you to Dr. Right because they have a friendly golf game
every week.

Physicians also have a natural tendency to refer patients to his or
her own hospital rather than to a nearby competitor, to get a new
program going, or even help one which is faltering at his or her
hospital despite the fact that the competitor may have a much higher
pregnancy rate. Remember: your goal is to have the best chance of
success, not necessarily to support the local hospital. It's also not
unusual for hospitals to allow their doctors investment opportunities,
which may then determine referral patterns. This practice is very
common with X-ray facilities. But, X-ray studies usually do not vary
that much in quality. You are looking for a service that *does* vary
markedly in quality.

Or, perhaps your doctor knows personally that Dr. Right is an
excellent physician and is also very personable and caring. Even so,
your doctor's Dr. Right could be your Dr. Wrong; so ask some
questions. A simple "Why are you referring me to Dr. Right?" may
provide important information. And even if the answer sounds good,
you are not finished with your investigation as you will see in a
moment.

• **PHYSICIAN–FRIEND**—The best possible referral source you can have,
if it's available, is a friend who is either a physician with firsthand
knowledge of the medical community or another health professional
who knows professionally and personally of the reputations of the
physicians you may wish to consider. This health professional–friend
as a friend has your best interests at heart and also has objective
information. In addition, by knowing you he or she can match you to

a physician based on both your medical and your emotional needs.

Here's a breakdown of the major referral sources ranked from best to worst, according to objectivity and to the extent that each is mindful of your needs.

1. Physician or health professional–friend
2. Your physician
3. Support groups
4. Friend who has had good results
5. Prestigious hospital referral service
6. County medical society
7. Classified telephone directory or advertising

INVESTIGATION OF RESOURCES

Armed with your list of potential providers, you are now ready to embark on the second part of the process, your investigation of these resources. We suggest you set up a chart with criteria to be determined along the vertical axis and the providers you are considering on the horizontal axis. You will find similar graphs in consumer magazines such as *Consumer Reports* for almost any item.

You can conduct this investigation either by telephone or in person. To save time, you may be able to eliminate some of the potential providers by telephone answers to your most important questions. Everyone's list of questions and concerns will be slightly different since we all have different needs. But there are some which will be universal.

Before we outline the most common areas of concern, a word of advice: It may be just as important to you *how* the questions are answered as what the actual answers are.

• When you call is the person you speak to friendly and helpful? Then, when you arrive at the office, are you treated as cheerfully as you were on the phone? Or do you find yourself suddenly in the domain of a Gestapolike office staff who coldly insist that you sign in, fill out the form, and take a seat? Remember, your experience with the office staff may a clue to the attitude of the physician in charge.

• Will this be a sit-down visit with your clothes on to obtain your history and discuss this huge investment in time, money, and your future you are about to make? In other words, does the first meeting occur in a relaxed atmosphere, or will you meet the physician or nurse coordinator for the first time only when you are bereft of the "protection" of your clothing, literally exposed in stirrups, already positioned in the role of dutiful, submissive patient? "Hey, wait a minute. Why are my feet in stirrups? I just came to ask questions!"

• What about the doctor's attitude? Regardless of where the consultation takes place, it's important that the doctor show genuine interest in your questions and concern about your problem. Do you have the doctor's undivided attention, or must you share it with frequent phone calls and interruptions from the front office? You should be mindful, of course, that the best physicians are often in high demand. So, more important, pay attention to *how* your questions are answered. Are there hints of resentment in the answers ("You don't need to concern yourself with that. That's my concern; *I'm* the doctor..."). Are the answers honest, straightforward, and clear, with facts to back them up? If the waiting room is packed, the doctor may be in a rush. You'll know this in advance of your meeting if you witness the doctor walking a patient down the hall and asking if she has any questions. So, be alert to indications of insincerity ("Don't worry, sweetheart. Everything will be just fine..."). Your Dr. Perfect will be the person who is concerned about you, interested in your problem, is honest, straightforward, one you can trust with your future, and someone who has the technical skills to treat your problem.

• One more point about attitude—this time yours. Greet the doctor with a positive outlook. Bivian Marr, our head nurse practitioner, is the one who does the initial intake history in our program. She finds that patients are frequently angry and hostile because they are frustrated with their infertility problem and give the impression that they may have been ripped off elsewhere. We suggest you begin your relationship with this potential Dr. Perfect by starting out with a clean slate. Tell him or her about yourself as succinctly as possible, leaving out extraneous material not relating to the present problem. Tell him or her who referred you. Don't become argumentative. Try not to put the doctor on the defensive. You're there to make an assessment, not score points in a debate. If you're nervous, that's okay. Remember, you're not the one who's auditioning, right?

TEN QUESTIONS

There are certain questions and concerns that we all would have regarding our entry into an ART program. There are also questions and concerns that may be unique to you as a couple. The following are just suggestions for you to include in your list of criteria on the graph you've already constructed.

1. SUCCESS RATE. The first consideration has got to be the success rate of the program. Close to 200 IVF programs were established in the United States by mid-1988. The pregnancy rates among these programs have been highly variable, with a number of teams having little or no success. Therefore, obtain a definite figure for success of the program you are investigating. Do not accept "average" success rates for *other* programs. Average success rates for other programs have no relationship to the success rate of the particular program you are investigating.

It is important for you to understand how success rates are calculated because there can be a wide variation in rates based on a program's experience just by juggling the figures. The success rate is calculated by creating a fraction and then converting it to a percentage. The top number of the fraction (the numerator) represents pregnancies, the bottom number (the denominator) represents procedures.

The fraction would look like this:

$$\frac{\text{PREGNANCIES}}{\text{PROCEDURES}} = \text{SUCCESS RATE}$$

But pregnancies could be any and all pregnancies, including:
- Biochemical pregnancies (a positive pregnancy test without ultrasound confirmation of a pregnancy)
- Clinical pregnancies that end as miscarriages or ectopic pregnancies
- Clinical pregnancies that go past twelve weeks
- Live births

Procedures could include any of the following:
- Patients undergoing stimulation
- Patients going on to egg retrieval
- Patients reaching embryo transfer

Using this fraction, you can see that if we use the greatest number of pregnancies possible, all pregnancies including biochemical, in the numerator and the smallest number of procedures, only patients reaching transfer, in the denominator, the success rate will be very high. (We do not feel that this gives an accurate indication of the success of a program.)

Let's look at an example. Here are the raw data representing one year's experience of an IVF program:

PROCEDURES   **RESULTS**
Stimulations—100   All pregnancies—20
Egg retrievals—90   Clinical pregnancies—13
Transfers—80   Live births—9

Here are the results, depending upon how these data are reported:

	All Pregnancies	Clinical	Live births
Stimulations	20%	13%	9%
Retrievals	22%	14%	10%
Transfers	25%	16%	11%

So you see that this IVF program, based on these raw data, could legitimately report success rates varying from 9 percent to 25 percent, depending upon what criteria were used. We feel that *the best reflection of the success of an IVF program is the rate of clinical pregnancy per egg retrieval.* By this method, our mythical IVF program should report a 14 percent success rate.

Ideally, the delivery rate of living babies is the most important numerator. This is because the definition of clinical pregnancy may vary among IVF programs, the level of miscarriage may be higher with poorer technique, and a live baby is really what you are striving for. But, using the "live-baby rate" is somewhat impractical since the rate of miscarriage may vary widely due to chance and there is an inherent nine-month delay from embryo transfer to delivery. Only well-established IVF programs can give a reasonably accurate "take-home-baby rate." In addition, by the time you obtain a rate based on "take-home" babies, it is based on techniques used and personnel involved over a year ago, a lengthy interval of time when considering ART procedures.

In the denominator we suggest egg retrievals rather than embryo transfer rate as the best reflection of IVF program quality because cases not reaching transfer could reflect deficiencies in egg retrieval or laboratory techniques and may give a falsely high success rate. The percentage of cancelled stimulations should also be examined because the success rate can be substantially influenced by allowing egg retrievals only when the results of stimulation are ideal. Therefore, for practical purposes we suggest:

$$\frac{\text{CLINICAL PREGNANCY}}{\text{EGG RETRIEVALS}} = \text{SUCCESS RATE}$$

Using this formula, you can use the figure of 10 percent clinical pregnancy rate per egg retrieval as the minimum level of performance to warrant confidence in an IVF program. Maximum rates have varied up to as high as 30 percent or more. For GIFT procedures, we consider 15 percent as a minimum to consider. Keep in mind that you are looking for excellence.

2. LEVEL OF ACTIVITY. You need to know how many cycles of IVF and GIFT are done by the physician in a year in order to gauge the significance of the quoted success rate. This does not mean that you should shy away from very small programs. On the contrary, many are excellent and afford you the individualization you may need. But, because of substantial variation based on chance alone, at least 100 cases are required to be able to quote a success rate that is a reasonably accurate reflection of the quality of the program. For example, in our program at AMI–South Bay Hospital we have had streaks of up to seven successful IVF cycles in a row. But we also experience occasional "dry" spells. Because of this, we always quote a success rate based on the last twelve months' experience reflecting our one to two hundred cases per year.

Not all programs report their total or annual experience. For example, in an editorial forum ("Medical Advertising: One Man's Opinion") in the American Fertility Society's newsletter *Fertility News,* Dr. J. Benjamin Younger from the University of Alabama–Birmingham criticizes a program that advertised "Our success rate is an impressive 30 percent, well above the national average." He states that this rate was calculated from four pregnancies among twelve patients. Review of the data in the congressional survey revealed no births from sixteen retrievals in 1987 and one live birth and three continuing pregnancies from thirty-one retrievals in 1988. The 30-percent success rate must have been culled from a very limited period of time within their total experience. If you calculate their success rate based on their total experience (only retrieval figures are available), still with a less than statistically significant number of cases, their success rate for 1987 and 1988 should have been cited as:

$$\frac{4 \text{ clinical pregnancies}}{47 \text{ retrievals}} = 9\%$$

If you consider only 1987, the calculation should be:

$$\frac{0 \text{ clinical pregnancies}}{16 \text{ retrievals}} = 0\%$$

If you take into account only 1988, the calculation would be as follows:

$$\frac{4 \text{ clinical pregnancies}}{31 \text{ retrievals}} = 13\%$$

3. STABILITY. A companion question will revolve around how long the program has been established. If they have not been doing ART for at least several years, inquire about how they learned these procedures. In order to learn the fine details that have proven successful through years of experience, these individuals must have prolonged and extensive experience with an established, successful program. How long has the team been together? Are the current members of the team the same people whose success rate they are quoting? There is some tendency for personnel in this sophisticated field to move from program to program. This is a complex process requiring a team composed of individuals with training and experience in pelvic surgery, reproductive endocrinology, andrology, and embryology. The absence of one of these key people could have a devastating effect on an otherwise excellent program. In some cases there actually may not be anyone who was even there when the quoted results were obtained.

4. SART MEMBERSHIP. All qualified programs should belong to the Society for Assisted Reproductive Technology (SART), a specialty group of the American Fertility Society (AFS). SART has set a minimum of forty completed cycles per year as the qualifying level of activity to participate as a member program. Additionally, the team must have experienced individuals at every level and must have had at least three live births from the program. Membership in SART assures you a minimum level of expertise and level of activity. There is, however, no assurance of a reasonable success rate, since achieving a certain rate is not a requirement for membership.

5. Cost. One of the most important considerations is the cost of whatever ART treatment you may need, and relative costs vary quite a bit. As determined by the congressional panel, the cost of an IVF cycle runs some $4000 to $7000 for each attempt. The largest variable will probably be geography, although centers in the same city may vary significantly. We certainly do not suggest that you "shop around" for the lowest price, but we do recommend that you fit cost into the equation relative to its importance to you. Do not compromise quality for cost, but if two of the programs you are considering are similar, cost may become the deciding factor. We currently have a couple in our program from a city about 300 miles away because their nearby program, although of similar quality, was much more expensive.

6. Qualifications of the Director. The director of the center or head physician of the team must be highly qualified. In addition to being board-certified in obstetrics and gynecology, he or she may also be boarded or have at least finished a special fellowship in reproductive endocrinology. This is an area of medicine, as we have stressed before, where intensive teamwork is required. But the responsibility for the success of the team lies with its director, and there is no substitute for a qualified and competent physician in this role. Get to know him or her. He or she is your Dr. Perfect.

7. Psychological Support. An experienced program should have readily available psychological support to optimize the couple's ability to cope with the stresses inherent in the process. Psychological issues can have a major impact on the success of an individual couple, since perseverance is a key to the ultimate chance of a pregnancy. Emotional stability and mutual support help a couple persist in their quest.

8. Flexibility. The flexibility of a physician's ideas and the program's protocols are very important. Is this the type of program that is going to fit you into a procedure because it is best for them, or will they individualize treatment? Do they try to push you into GIFT because *they* are having difficulty with their embryo transfer technique? Will they individualize the stimulation protocol to vary the dose and timing of drugs based on your needs, or is everyone treated the same? Our bias is toward individualization.

9. METHOD OF RETRIEVAL. How are the eggs retrieved? At this time almost everyone is using transvaginal ultrasound-guided egg retrieval. However, there are still some holdouts for laparoscopy. The ultrasound technique, described in Chapter 7, utilizes sedation rather than anesthesia and requires less recovery time. Patients who have experienced both uniformly prefer the ultrasound technique. The only drawback to ultrasound aspiration is that the diagnostic and therapeutic aspects of laparoscopy are lost. In some individual cases there may be aspects important enough to justify the additional expense and risk of laparoscopy. Of course, with GIFT and ZIFT, laparoscopy is required.

10. ALL TREATMENT METHODS AVAILABLE. A quality operation should have all current methods of treatment available. An example might be embryo freezing. By limiting the number of fresh embryos transferred to three or four, the risk of multiple pregnancy can be better controlled. Freezing additional embryos can reduce costs considerably by allowing multiple embryo transfer procedures from one stimulation and retrieval. In some women, the uterus may not be receptive in the stimulated cycle. For example, Patty, whom you met in Chapter 1, became pregnancy only after a frozen embryo transfer.

ADDITIONAL QUESTIONS

You may have some questions addressing your particular concerns such as age, distance, or prior surgery. Here are some examples:

Doctor, I'm forty-one years old. I know that you generally have very good results, but what are your results with women my age?

We live about 400 miles up the coast. Since it would be so expensive for me to travel or stay here, can my doctor there start my medications?

I had my tubes tied by Band-aid surgery. The other doctor told me that surgery to repair my tubes would be better than IVF.

My friend had some bleeding after her eggs were picked up. Do you ever have complications?

Now, there you have tools you'll need for finding Dr. Perfect. Don't be afraid to use them. Keep reminding yourself that having your baby is well worth whatever effort it takes. While you may not find Dr. Perfect, we believe that you'll come a lot closer to him or her than the countless others who will rely mainly on factors that have little to do with the quality of care they will receive.

nine

A Lifetime of Hope In About Thirty Days

It's amazing how much of what we do is timed according to the number of days it takes the moon to revolve around the earth. That interval of time is 29.25 days, approximately one month. It is usually how often we pay our bills, the period of time on one page of a calendar, and the basic unit we use to rent an apartment or pay our mortgage. People see the time frame of thirty days as significant, often choosing it to reach a particular goal. For example, in advertisements on the back of comic books and magazines in the late 1950s bodybuilder Charles Atlas boasted, "In just 30 days I can make you a man." A book promised *Thirty Days to a More Powerful Vocabulary*.

We could have titled this chapter "In Just Thirty Days We Can Make You a Baby," but this concept does not agree with our outlook that it is the *couple* who makes the baby; we just help. But it is true that all of the ART procedures do encompass an approximate thirty-day interval. This is simply because these procedures are coordinated to the menstrual cycle, which averages twenty-eight to thirty days. Having taken hundreds of couples through these procedures, we know that they are investing not only their money and time in this process but also all of their life's hopes and dreams in the events that will take place in the next thirty days.

THE PATIENT'S PERSPECTIVE

If you are planning to go through an IVF, GIFT, or related procedure, you want to know what actually happens on a day-to-day basis. Although we can outline from the IVF team's point of view what each day involves, we enlisted the services of Cheryl Scruggs, one of our IVF patients, to provide you with a look at each day's activities through the eyes of a typical patient.

Before we start, we want you to understand how Cheryl and Jeff Scruggs came to need IVF. Cheryl, then twenty-seven, was a sales representative for Konica Business Machines. Jeff, twenty-eight, was a sales representative for the children's clothing company Oshkosh B'Gosh. (They both felt that there was a certain irony that Jeff was in the children's clothing business while they were unable to have a child.) Their struggle with infertility was slightly unusual in that they had tried to conceive for only nine months before quickly discovering their problem. Because of the severity of the problem they immediately opted for IVF. Most other couples struggle for many years before reaching IVF or GIFT.

Cheryl had come in for a routine annual examination and had expressed her concern that she had been trying to get pregnant for nine months and nothing was happening. She remembers that "in my heart, I knew something was wrong." Because of her concern, she was started on a basal body temperature chart and a semen analysis was obtained on Jeff (it was normal). Her BBT showed that she was ovulating. But a hysterosalpingogram done on September 8, 1986, showed that both tubes were closed and, in fact, looked as if she had a hydrosalpinx on each side. In order to determine the exact nature of her tubal problem and what it would take to repair it, she underwent a laparoscopy. On October 10, 1986, her worst fears were confirmed. After the laparoscopy, Jeff was told Cheryl's tubes were indeed closed. In addition, the fimbria at the end of both tubes were destroyed and each tube ended in a blind dilated sac. The extent of tubal damage and surrounding scar tissue indicated a poor prognosis for surgical repair. He was told that tubal microsurgery would yield only a 10 percent chance of pregnancy in her case. After the laparoscopy, she was too groggy to really discuss the findings, and an appointment was made for several days later to discuss the situation thoroughly.

I remember driving home from surgery and no one had told me what they had found. Jeff said that we would talk about it after I got some rest. "No," I said, "tell me the results NOW!" Jeff, with tears in his eyes, said that my tubes looked really bad. They were blocked and scarred and basically nothing could be done to fix the problem. He said we could try surgery to fix the tubes or attempt in vitro fertilization. He said that the doctor felt that surgery was not my best option since there was only a 10 percent chance it would work. I was devastated to think I could never have my own child. My mom was so fertile and popped babies out right and left. How could I have problems?

Several days later, the options were discussed with Cheryl and Jeff. Those options were tubal repair, IVF, or adoption. The best option appeared to them to be IVF. They were young, Jeff had a good semen analysis, and their only problem was the tubal obstruction. Statistically, IVF had a higher success rate than tubal repair. Adoption was not an option they would select at this time.

Cheryl was in a hurry to get started, but there were obstacles. At that time, there was an eighteen- to twenty-four-month waiting list before a patient could enter the program.

I was very impatient because we wanted to get started. I felt deep in my heart that once we started we would reach our dream of having a baby. We kept a positive attitude and feel that this can make the odds better for success. We waited approximately nine months. I called the IVF center almost every day. The nurse-coordinator thought I was neurotic and totally obsessed.

Cheryl's persistence paid off. The program was just at the point of changing its method of retrieval to a simpler technique that could become routine for most patients. Cheryl immediately volunteered for the transvaginal ultrasound method and by June 1987 was started in the program.

THIRTY DAYS HATH SEPTEMBER, APRIL, JUNE, AND IVF...

In taking you through a "typical" cycle, we will be using the stimulation protocol, retrieval, and transfer procedures along with instructions used at the AMI–South Bay Hospital In Vitro Fertilization Center. Obviously, if you go through IVF at another center or choose another procedure altogether, you may have a slightly different experience. That does not mean that our way is right and theirs is wrong, or vice versa. As we've said before, there are many different ways of doing these procedures. So, if you experience differences, don't be alarmed.

With that caveat, let us begin. Since we use leuprolide (Lupron) to supress the ovary, our Day 1 is not the first day of the menstrual period. It is when the patient first comes in to start Lupron. This will be about one week after ovulation as determined by detection of the LH surge by a urine test or by a temperature chart. We have patients with open tubes use a barrier method of contraception since they will be using a medication before we could determine if they were pregnant.

Day 1

Six days after the rise of the temperature is detected, the patient comes into the center with her first morning urine specimen. The urine is tested for a form of progesterone that indicates that ovulation has taken place. A vaginal ultrasound will be done to ensure that the pelvic structures are normal. No preparation is necessary for the vaginal ultrasound. The bladder does not even need to be full for this type of scan. There is minimal discomfort.

If the urine test is positive and the ultrasound is normal, the patient is instructed in the technique of injecting the Lupron. It is given subcutaneously (into the fatty tissue under the skin) through a small, painless needle.

By June 1987 I was totally obsessed and overly anxious. Although I was about to start at a time when they were getting close to their summer break, I decided to go ahead anyway. I pushed them into letting me start. I felt as if I was up against a deadline to completely finish the process before they closed down.

Days 2 Through Day 9

All that is required during this period is to take the daily injection of Lupron in the morning and wait for Day 10 along with the start of the next menstrual period.

Day 10

If the patient's menstrual period has begun, she returns to the center for an ultrasound scan and estrogen level. The ultrasound is to detect any abnormalities in the pelvis or residual cysts and other structures from the previous cycle that may interfere with the stimulation. The estrogen level is supposed to be suppressed by the

Lupron. So, if the scan is normal and the estrogen low, the patient is ready to begin her stimulation. If her period does not start, the scan and estrogen level will be delayed until the menstrual flow begins. If her estrogen is not supressed or if cysts are seen on the ultrasound, she will return at four-day intervals until everything is right. But for most patients Day 10 happens on the tenth day.

> Because my cycle is normally so long, I was on Lupron longer than usual. I got very impatient and anxious, which I feel slowed my body's natural cycle and therefore made the process longer. I did not make it this time to the Pergonal. I was dropped because my period was so delayed and they could not have possibly finished my cycle before they were scheduled to close for their summer vacation. Actually, Jeff felt it was better that we stopped then because I was really not in the right frame of mind.
>
> I was very upset, almost mad at them. They told me I would have to wait until September to try again. Another three months; I couldn't believe it! I knew it would be the longest three months of my entire life. That night I cried and cried. We went to the support group sponsored by the center, but we didn't feel that it was to our benefit. Believe it or not, many of the people in the group were more emotional than I was. We actually felt that our emotions were in control. That summer went fast. We took a trip back east to see our families. We also spent a lot of time at the beach. All I wanted to do was get started. I knew it would work.

On Day 10 the daily injection of Pergonal begins. It is usually given between 7:00 P.M. to 9:00 P.M. It is generally too difficult for the woman to give to herself, so her husband will usually give it or make alternate arrangements. The routine dosage is two or three ampules injected deeply into the muscle of the buttocks. If the total daily dose of Pergonal is more than three ampules, we prefer to divide it into two injections: one in the morning, the other in the evening. In addition, the Lupron is continued each morning, but at half the original dose. So there may be up to three injections a day until the patient is ready for the HCG.

> Before starting my second attempt, I had to start my period. As I expected, it was six days late. I couldn't wait to call the center even though I was scared to start the process. It was starting to bother me that all of our friends and family were having babies. It was now hard for me to be around babies. I really never felt jealous of these people. It just made me want one even more so. I had not accepted the fact that we may never have children of our own, or that our only option might be to adopt. I felt guilty because I blamed myself for not

being able to conceive. Jeff is a very supportive person and always told me it was "our" problem, not mine.

When I called the IVF Center, they told me to come in October tenth to start the Lupron. They taught me how to inject the Lupron into my thigh or abdomen. I really didn't look forward to the shots, but I knew that every injection was getting us closer and closer to possibly having our own baby. I would have done anything to have a baby, no matter what I had to sacrifice.

It was a strange sensation feeling the needle just below the skin and actually seeing the medication make a little bubble. With the Lupron, it was very important to place the needle just below the skin, not into the muscle. The spot where I placed the needle would swell up, get very hot and would itch for about 30 minutes. I also had hot flashes and would perspire. While taking the Lupron, I felt somewhat tired, but not depressed. I was a little moody, so Jeff would rub my back, hug me or do whatever would make me comfortable.

Days 11 Through 14 (Starting Pergonal)

After the visit on Day 10 or so to confirm suppression of the ovary, no visits to the center are necessary for five days. The patient continues to take her regimen of Pergonal and Lupron injections and can carry on normal daily activity.

The Pergonal scared me a little mainly because of the size of the needle, which was about one inch long. Jeff had to administer the Pergonal once a day at 7 P.M. into my hip. I dreaded the shot because it did hurt some. But I was willing to do anything to achieve a pregnancy.

Jeff tried to make it a comical situation. He'd say, "Okay, honey. Pull your pants down and bend over. It's time for your shot." Jeff was a pro. He put the needle in fast and I barely felt it go in. The first couple of times he didn't place it in the right spot in my hip, which would cause my leg to ache for a couple of hours. We called the IVF Center and they made us come in and take another lesson in where to place the needle. After that, we had no problems.

Day 15

By this time five doses of Pergonal have been given and it is time to return to the center to see how the follicles are progressing. A vaginal ultrasound will be done and then the dose of Pergonal will be adjusted, depending on the response of the follicles. If there is little activity, the Pergonal will likely be increased. If the ultrasound shows many follicles developing, the Pergonal may be lowered. The doctor will get the first indication of the adequacy of the stimulation at this point. The Lupron is continued at the same dose no matter what the findings on ultrasound. An appointment will be made to return in from one to three days, depending on the response.

> The Pergonal made me even more tired. At this point I was seeing the doctor every day for an ultrasound. I responded very well to the Pergonal. Every ultrasound showed more and more eggs. I was very excited, yet felt nervous. I just prayed that all would go well.

Day 16

Assuming we are dealing with the average patient, no visit would be required on this day, but the Pergonal and Lupron would be given.

Day 17 (The Day of HCG)

Seven days of Pergonal have been given, and by this time it should be possible to evaluate the response. Some patients will get their HCG injection on this day to trigger ovulation. Others will receive the HCG any time within the next three to four days. This is the point at which the determination to continue the cycle or to "drop" it will usually be made. If there are not enough follicles developing or one follicle is far more developed than the others, a decision to stop the process may be made. An estradiol level obtained as the follicles approach maturity could indicate that there are too many small follicles producing an excess of estrogen. Rarely, this could make continuing the cycle too dangerous and force the process to be stopped. With the use of Lupron to suppress the ovary prior to the use of the hMG, we have experienced a dropout rate of about 10 percent, compared to about 30 percent prior to the use of Lupron. The decision on which day to give the HCG is based on correlating follicle size and number with the estradiol level. Generally, it would be given anywhere from Day 17 to Day 21, with the average patient receiving her HCG on Day 19.

The most important features about the HCG injection are that it be given *precisely* at the time instructed and that it be given correctly. Since ovulation becomes increasingly common after thirty-six hours following the HCG injection, the retrieval will be timed to occur 34.5 hours after the HCG. If the HCG is given too early, the follicles might ovulate spontaneously. If it is given too late, the follicles might not be optimally ready for retrieval. If the injection is not given in its entirety, the lower blood levels achieved might compromise the cycle.

Cheryl received her HCG after only seven doses of Pergonal. (The average patient receives the HCG after ten days of Pergonal.) On that day, November 4, 1987, she had eighteen follicles measured with several small ones noted. Her estradiol level was 2168. Because of the large number of follicles present and the estradiol over 2000, it was felt that the Pergonal stimulation should go no further because a very high estrogen level may have a detrimental effect on implantation. She was scheduled to receive her HCG at precisely 9:00 P.M. and the ultrasound retrieval was scheduled for 7:30 A.M. on November 6, 1987.

> We had plans to go to dinner with some friends at 7 P.M. We were only going five minutes away from home, but did not want to chance not being home by nine. We took the HCG shot with us. Our friends whom we were meeting had also been through IVF. They were successful with quadruplets (in Dr. Meldrum's program—the first in the country through IVF) and fully understood what we were going through.
>
> When we arrived at the restaurant, we explained to the hostess that it was vital to us that I have this shot at exactly 9 P.M. and asked if they had a place we could use for a few minutes. We sat down for dinner and at 9 P.M. they ushered us into their food storage room. When we entered, we burst out with laughter. Around us were shelves with box after box of ketchup, salt, bacon bits, etc. I told Jeff that we needed to lock the door, but there was no lock. So, I took off my high heels and pulled my pants down. Jeff was laughing so hard that he didn't think he would be able to give me the shot. I was afraid that someone would open the door and see me with my pants down. Sure enough, just as Jeff was about to hit me with the needle, the door flew open. It shut immediately and all we could hear was laughter and apologies. Jeff finally gave me the shot and we returned to our table in hysterics.

Day 18 (The Day After HCG)

The patients return to the center for:
- Ultrasound to check on the status of the follicles
- Blood sample to make sure that the estradiol does not drop dramatically, which would indicate a problem with follicle development
- Brief history and physical examination in anticipation of the retrieval procedure the next day

Perhaps the most important feature of this visit is the thorough explanation of the retrieval procedure along with its expectations and potential complications. We go through the entire technical procedure, along with information about sedation or anesthesia and expectations of results, then discuss what will be done with the eggs after the retrieval. This is a good time for the couple to ask questions to relieve any fears or concerns they may have. It is important to have all of the important decisions regarding embryo freezing made and all consents signed by this time. Even if general anesthesia is not given, we advise not having anything to eat or drink after midnight.

Day 19 (The Retrieval)

The patient is admitted to the center about an hour and a half before the scheduled time of the retrieval. An IV is started in her arm and some fluids and an antibiotic are given. An injection of a narcotic is given intramuscularly. She is then wheeled on a stretcher to the procedure room.

She is placed in a position similar to that of a pelvic examination, with her legs supported by stirrups. Additional sedation in the form of a tranquilizer is given slowly through the IV. The nurse washes the area outside the vagina with an antiseptic solution and then inserts a catheter into the bladder to keep the bladder empty during the procedure. She then washes out the inside of the vagina with the antiseptic. The washing of the vagina can be uncomfortable, but by this time most patients are fairly well sedated and tolerate it without too much discomfort.

The doctor washes out the antiseptic from the vagina with a special sterile solution. The area around the vagina is surrounded by sterile drapes. A sterile plastic cover is placed over the ultrasound instrument; a tube to guide the needle is attached and it is placed into the vagina exactly as it had been when the follicles were being monitored. The collection system is tested and the procedure is ready to begin. Additional amounts of narcotic are given through the IV as needed. We also find it helpful to have the patient listen to her favorite music through a set of headphones. She can bring her own tapes or we will provide her favorite radio station. Most patients talk to the staff during the procedure and many follow the count of eggs retrieved and can find out the quality of the eggs from the person screening them.

With the ultrasound visualizing the follicles, the needle is placed by means of the guide through the vaginal wall and into the nearest follicle in the ovary. The passage of the needle through the vaginal wall and into the ovary is the only part of the procedure that most patients feel. Once the needle is in the ovary and moved from one follicle to another, the majority of patients feel little or nothing. Each follicle is aspirated and may be flushed several times until the egg is found. The fluid returns through the needle and tubing into a test tube. This tube is passed to a team member who labels the tube and quickly places it into the incubator, which is maintained at body temperature with a special 5 percent carbon dioxide atmosphere. The screener pours the fluid into a small dish and examines the contents under a microscope until the egg is found. Mature eggs are usually visible with the naked eye because of a halo of transluscent tissue around them. Any comments regarding the quality of the egg will be noted and it is transferred to a test tube containing a nutrient medium for incubation.

The procedure is repeated until all the follicles on each side have been asprated and flushed. The pelvis is then scanned to be sure that there are no additional follicles present and that there is no evidence of bleeding. The drapes are removed, the patient's legs are taken out of the stirrups, and she will be observed in the center for two to four hours. During this time, her blood pressure and pulse will be monitored and she will be given some fluids and medication for pain or nausea, if needed.

> We arrived at the hospital about 7 A.M. to prepare for the egg retrieval. They gave me a shot of Demerol, which I had an immediate reaction to. I broke out in a cold sweat, felt nauseous, and my blood pressure went down. I was getting sleepy and light-headed. Jeff was by my side during the preparation. He held my hand, kissed me, and was very comforting. I was scared, yet excited. During the procedure I really couldn't feel much except when the medication started to wear off. Then I could feel a tug in my ovaries as if they were extracting something. They got 23 eggs! Everyone was so excited. They took me to the recovery room and said I'd go home at 2 P.M. But I was extremely sick to my stomach and couldn't stop vomiting. I ended up staying until 6:30 P.M.

After the egg retrieval is completed, it is time for collection of the semen specimen. It is suggested that the last prior ejaculation be about two to four days before the retrieval. The specimen is obtained by masturbation into a sterile nontoxic container and washed with nutrient medium in the laboratory. Approximately 50,000 sperm are added to each egg which, by now, has incubated for several hours. In the event of a male factor problem, up to 500,000 sperm may be added to each egg.

> As they wheeled me to recovery, they asked Jeff to collect his specimen. He was somewhat embarrassed, but was actually used to giving specimens as he previously had sperm counts, antibody tests, and the hamster test.

Following the retrieval, medications are limited to acetaminophen (Tylenol) or codeine if there is any discomfort. A light diet and rest are recommended. The only other task remaining on this day is to begin progesterone injections, which are given deep in the muscle each evening starting the night of the retrieval. The dose varies and is proportional to the estradiol level on the day of HCG administration. The couple goes to sleep at home as their eggs and sperm are uniting in the laboratory.

Day 20

Early in the morning the eggs are checked for the first time for indications that fertilization has taken place. Each egg is examined under the microscope looking for the two pronuclei indicating that genetic material from only one sperm and one egg is present. The occasional egg that may have been fertilized with more than one sperm (polyspermic) will be screened out and discarded. Eggs that did not fertilize will be reinseminated. If there are more embryos than can be transferred during this cycle, some extra embryos will be frozen at this pronuclear stage. A call will be made to the couple giving them the information regarding the status of their embryos and final arrangements will be made for the time of the embryo transfer the next day. The second dose of progesterone is given at 7:00 P.M.

> On Saturday, November 7, we called to find out how many eggs had fertilized. We were delighted to learn that 15 had fertilized. One had been fertilized by more than one sperm, so we had 14 embryos to work with.

Day 21 (Embryo Transfer)

This is the day of the embryo transfer. The patient may have a light breakfast and will take an antibiotic tablet. We recommend limiting fluids as we prefer she not have to get up to urinate for the three hours of rest after the transfer. The transfer procedure is actually quite easy for the patient. She is given a dose of Valium so that she is relaxed. She is placed in the position for a pelvic examination with her legs supported by stirrups. Meanwhile, the embryos are being examined in the laboratory under the microscope and evaluated for the number of cells, consistency of size of each cell, and the presence of fragments of cells within the embryo. The best embryos have the following characteristics:

- Greatest number of cells
- Uniformity of size of cells
- Absence of fragmentation

When the best embryos have been selected for transfer, they are placed in a dish. The plastic catheter has been molded to the shape of the uterine cavity as determined at the time of the trial transfer before this cycle began. It is rinsed with medium. The incubator is rolled into the transfer room, which is quiet and has had the lights dimmed. A speculum is inserted into the vagina and the cervix is washed with medium.

The husband is then asked if he wishes to look at the embryos. He usually agrees. This is a very emotional moment as he looks at the three or four embryos consisting of only a few cells which may become his offspring. The embryos are drawn up into the catheter attached to a very accurate syringe and passed to the physician. It is up to the physician to carefully thread this catheter containing the embryos up through the cervix and into the uterus just a fraction of an inch away from the top of the cavity. The whole process depends on these embryos being deposited gently in the right place, allowing them the best chance of implanting.

About one minute after the embryos have been expelled the catheter is withdrawn and checked for retained embryos. If the catheter is empty, the speculum is removed and the patient is placed head down on her stomach or back, depending on the position of the uterus. She is allowed to rest for fifteen minutes before being transferred to a room where she will stay at bedrest for an additional three hours. She will go home and continue bedrest for the next forty-eight hours. She will continue receiving progesterone each day.

We arrived at the IVF Center at 9:30 A.M. They put me in a hospital gown and gave me Valium. I was nervous and felt cold. The best part was that Jeff could come in the room during the transfer. I started to cry. I'm not sure why. Maybe it was just to relieve the pressure because I knew that this was "it." Would it work? We went into the quiet, dark room. Jeff was holding my hand and in my other hand was my rosary. Although I am not a practicing Catholic any more, I have had that rosary since I was a kid and I felt I wanted it with me. I was praying and smiling.

They brought the incubator in with the embryos in it. Jeff looked in the microscope and saw the four embryos. He said that it was an unbelievable feeling. He was possibly looking at his future child or even children. All the embryos were four or five cells, which meant they were healthy and strong. They placed them into my uterus very carefully. There was no pain. After the transfer they took me to a hospital room where I had to lie on my stomach with the head of the bed lower than my feet for three hours. I was unable to sleep and had no entertainment or radio. My head kept sliding into the headboard and my neck was killing me. Jeff went home for a while and came back to get me. I went home and was instructed to stay in bed for two days.

Days 22 and 23

These two days are spent at home on complete bedrest. The only injection required is the dose of progesterone which will be given at about 7:00 P.M.

I couldn't do anything except go to the bathroom. No showers, no walking around, no cooking—nothing! Jeff brought all my meals upstairs and basically waited on me hand and foot. I read magazines, watched television, and slept.

Days 24 Through Day 35

Following the two days of bedrest, normal activity is allowed. We recommend against any strenuous physical activity, exercise, or sports. We also advise against intercourse or even other stimulation to orgasm. We really don't know what effect activity has after the transfer, but after going through so much, it is better to be cautious. The progesterone injections are continued daily.

I was able to get up, but was supposed to take it easy. I went back to work the following Monday, but for only half-days. But, more than anything else, I worried. We had been through so much that if it failed, I now knew that I would be very upset.

Day 36 (The Pregnancy Test)

This is it! Years of trying, testing, and treatment all culminate in one test this day. Two weeks following the transfer, she returns to the center for the pregnancy test. Actually, the pregnancy test can be done at any reliable medical laboratory. But if the patients live close to the center, we request that they do this test at the center, where we can share the news—good or bad—with them. The beta-HCG is a blood test that can be done in less than an hour. Some couples wait in the waiting room for the results. Some can't stand the suspense and go out for a walk while the test is being done. Some couples come together; some women come and face the news alone.

If the test is positive, there are usually tears of joy. These tears are not always limited to the couple. The members of the IVF team, even those not directly involved in medical activities, share the intense joy of the successful patients. The couple will be told that the positive pregnancy test is a first step toward their goal and that there are still some hurdles to encounter. We offer our congratulations and give them early pregnancy instructions. (We discuss those instructions and the special concerns in an IVF pregnancy in Chapter 10.)

If the test is negative, there are also tears shed, but these are the tears of bitter disappointment. Some patients want to discuss the technical aspects of their cycle at this time. Some express their disappointment and leave. Most, however, express surprisingly little outward emotion at this time. Perhaps they expected bad news, or perhaps they prefer to express their grief in private. In any event, we recommend to them that they return in a couple of weeks to air their feelings, review their cycle to see if any aspects of the process can be improved, and to discuss their plans for the future.

The pregnancy test was scheduled for November 22, 1987. I was already feeling a little sick, my breasts were tender, but I really believed that it was all in my head.

The night before the pregnancy test we went to dinner with our neighbors. When we went home they hugged us and by then we were all crying. We could feel their hope and concern. They wished us well. Earlier that week I had gone to lunch with my friend Jill, and she kept saying that she knew I was pregnant. I didn't want to get my hopes up because I was scared to death that it may not have worked. The two weeks after the transfer seemed like an eternity. Jeff and I talked a lot about the procedure and what would happen if it failed. When we got to the center, they called me in to take my blood. They asked me how I felt, if my breasts hurt, and if I was nauseous. When I said yes, they said those were good signs. They told us that it would take about 45 minutes. By this time I was really keyed up. My heart was beating fast and I didn't know if I could last another 45 minutes. We decided to go for a walk to kill some time. Jeff was nervous, too, but he tried not to show it. We made small talk while holding hands tightly. Secretly, I think we were both praying. After the walk, we went back into the center and sat down impatiently. My legs were shaking. We saw Minda, who had screened and cared for our eggs, come out of the lab to talk to us. I could see that she had tears in her eyes. My immediate thought was that it didn't work. She shook her head, "Yes, you are pregnant." Jeff and I immediately burst into tears and held each other tight. I was, for once, speechless. Our dream had come true.

They then told us that my pregnancy hormone level was so high they were sure it was more than one. We were ecstatic because we actually wanted twins. We immediately went home and told all of our neighbors and called all of our family and closest friends. There were many tears of joy.

Day 37 and Beyond

In thirty days, more or less, we have couples who must bear the disappointment of failure and figure out where to go from there. Will another IVF cycle be worthwhile? Will there soon be some scientific breakthrough which will make their chances better? Will their marriage even survive this disappointment?

On the other hand, we have couples who are about to embark on a journey through the next nine months which will, if all goes well, give them the child they have so longed for.

Two weeks later I was scheduled for my first ultrasound to see how many babies I had. During those two weeks, we pondered the thought of twins or triplets. Twins sounded wonderful; triplets maybe more than we could handle. The ultrasound showed twins.

Cheryl's pregnancy went quite smoothly. On July 18, 1988, she delivered twin girls by caesarean section because both babies were coming feet first. Brittany Marie weighed 6 pounds 11 ounces and Lauren Nicole tipped the scales at 6 pounds 7 ounces. From the start, Cheryl and Jeff considered their IVF cycle their "science project." They kept their sense of humor throughout this difficult period. They were fortunate enough to have the support of their family, friends, and, most important, each other. They both feel that it was this mutual support that sustained them.

...GIFT, ZIFT, PROST, AND TE(S)T

These procedures differ from IVF in that an operation is required both to retrieve eggs and to transfer egg and sperm into the fallopian tube in GIFT, and to transfer various-stage embryos in ZIFT, PROST, and TE(S)T. The stimulation phase will be similar to what we described in IVF. In ZIFT, PROST, and TE(S)T the egg retrieval will be identical to IVF. With GIFT, the laparoscopy is performed on Day 19, the day of retrieval. In the case of ZIFT, PROST, and TE(S)T, it is done on Day 20 or 21, depending on the stage of embryos to be transferred.

The patient is admitted to the hospital in the day surgery area. An IV is started and the anesthesiologist discusses the anesthetic options with her. These would include:

- Epidural, in which local anesthetic is injected near the spinal column. It numbs the tissues below the waist while the patient remains awake but can be sedated.
- General anesthesia, in which the patient is given an intravenous medication to induce sleep, and then gas is administered through a tube placed into the lungs to reach a deep level of anesthesia.

If the general anesthesia is chosen, the patient's abdomen is washed and drapes are placed around the lower abdomen before the anesthetic is given in order to reduce the period of time the eggs are exposed to the anesthetic. With the epidural, the anesthetic is administered first, since very little of the medication gets into the bloodstream.

A small incision is made in the lower margin of the navel. A thin needle is introduced into the abdominal cavity and a gas is put in to allow the surrounding tissues to fall away from the pelvic organs. The sheath for the telescope is then placed through the same incision and the pelvis is observed. Smaller incisions are made in the lower part of the abdomen for the other instruments to hold and move structures, to aspirate the follicles, or to place gametes into the fallopian tube.

If GIFT is being done, the ovary is brought into view and each follicle is punctured, aspirated, and flushed with medium until the egg is found. The eggs are identified, the quality is assessed, and those suitable for transfer are chosen. With GIFT, usually three to four eggs with 100,000 sperm are placed into the better-looking fallopian tube. While the eggs and sperm are being prepared, the pelvis is inspected for any abnormalities such as endometriosis. If any endometriosis is found, it can be cauterized. The sperm and eggs are then drawn up into a catheter placed through one of the incisions and guided about 3 centimeters into the tube. The eggs and sperm are expelled, the catheter is removed, all instruments are withdrawn, and the incisions are closed. After several hours of recovery, the patient may go home and, after recuperation, may engage in light activity for the next two weeks, until the pregnancy test. She will also be taking daily progesterone injections.

In some cases combined IVF/GIFT may be done. If some of the eggs are less mature, they can be allowed to further develop before the sperm are added. Then if embryos form, a transcervical transfer can be done two days later, as with IVF.

In the case of ZIFT, PROST, or TE(S)T, the eggs will be retrieved as described for IVF. They would be transferred during the next day or two, depending upon what stage embryo was to be transferred. One disadvantage is the need for two separate procedures for retrieval and transfer. This increases cost, discomfort, and risk. On the other side of the balance, initial small studies have indicated a higher success rate.

One of the most poignant accounts of a patient going through a ZIFT procedure was provided by Anne Taylor Fleming, the noted writer and media commentator, in a March 15, 1989, column in *The New York Times*. She described her second attempt at ZIFT at what she describes as "one of California's leading edge infertility clinics."

> So I am—or was—a pioneer of sorts, pregnant with optimism throughout the two weeks of fertility drugs before the procedure, and the two weeks after as you hold your breath for fear of dislodging any embryos that might have nestled within. It is suspended time; you live backward, taking inventory of the decisions that brought you to this point, and forward, imagining your barren years ahead. Your womb seems to be calling you to account, making you heed its emptiness. "At last I've got your attention," it seems to be saying. "Where have you been all these years?" But along with the deliberations and discomforts, there are incredible highs. The process is akin to being in a demonic love affair, when the pull and punishment of the flesh are irresistible. When I found they had retrieved 11 eggs from my ovaries, I was elated. How could I miss? But, by nightfall, I was in despair: What if none of the eggs fertilized: what if on the most basic level my husband and I were hopelessly incompatible, our sperm and eggs unwilling to conduct their extra-corporeal courtship; what if by morning we had no zygotes?
>
> The nurse called early to say we indeed had zygotes. Four eggs had fertilized. "Come get them," she said, and my heart leaped at the invitation. I dressed carefully and washed my hair, as if I were about to meet somebody special. Would I be able to hold onto one or any of them; would they continue to divide and grow inside me? Knowing the ZIFT odds, I was hopeful. No, that's not strong enough: I was crazed with hope as they put me to sleep, made a tiny slit in my navel and through a catheter dropped three of my embryos (the fourth was frozen for a future attempt) into my one good fallopian tube. All those embryos had to do is migrate down to my waiting womb. What could stop them now?
>
> Something did, some something. My embryos didn't take hold; they vanished. When that was confirmed, two weeks to the day after the procedure had been performed, I myself vanished for a while into a fetal curl of grief. This was hardly a death, not even a miscarriage, just a noncarriage.

So what's next? For me my remaining frozen embryo. It (he, she?) will be thawed and inseminated [sic] into my uterus in another month or so, after my body recovers from this last assault. . . . Out beyond that I can try another ZIFT. The woman who went through it the same day I did is pregnant. With clenched teeth, I rejoice for her.

How many rounds do I have left and how far am I willing to go before I give up or consider another course like adoption? I don't know.

SUCCESS AND FAILURE

The most intense thirty or so days in the lives of these couples is now over. There can be only two possible results: success in the form of a baby in the next nine months; or failure by means of a negative pregnancy test, miscarriage, ectopic pregnancy, or other obstetrical problem.

The couples who do not conceive have to deal with the bitterness of not having the opportunity of achieving their goal this time. They face an uncertain future and a decision of whether to try again, give up the fight, or go in a different direction such as adoption.

Fortunately, for most, a second, third, or fourth attempt will have a similar chance as the first. In fact, there is no single factor more important to ultimate success than having repeated attempts. Does this sound familiar? Yes, persistence is the key to success.

For some couples special problems may have been recognized during the first attempt. In Chapter 11 we will discuss the role egg and sperm donors can play in overcoming problems with the production of normal healthy eggs or with fertilization. For some, new experimental procedures may be possible (Chapter 12).

Those who are pregnant will enjoy the sweetness of their success. The positive pregnancy test, of course, is not the end point, but merely the beinning of the pregnancy that will lead them to their ultimate goal, a healthy baby. Yet there may be some potential hazards along the way; these we discuss in Chapter 10.

ten

And Baby Makes Three ... or Four

T he key question to be answered for those who are pregnant as the result of an ART procedure is whether these pregnancies are at greater risk than those conceived in the usual manner. Of course, multiple pregnancies—there is a stronger likelihood when ovulatory drugs and ART procedures are used—are more risky in general. But, aside from the increased risk from multiple pregnancy, are there additional perils for the ART pregnancy? We will explore this issue after we give you some basic advice.

CONGRATULATIONS, YOUR PREGNANCY TEST IS POSITIVE

Those are the words you want to hear, but they do not necessarily reflect the ultimate goal you want to achieve. The positive pregnancy test is just one step, albeit a very important one, along the way. Yet many couples misinterpret the positive pregnancy test as a sign that they have achieved their final goal. Actually, one of three outcomes can occur following the positive pregnancy test.

BIOCHEMICAL PREGNANCY. This is a situation in which fertilization has taken place, the embryo implants and starts to produce one of the pregnancy hormones (HCG), but something goes wrong with the implantation or the pregnancy fails to develop. A weakly positive pregnancy test indicates the presence of a pregnancy although no evidence of a pregnancy can be detected by ultrasound. The HCG level gradually declines to zero without any clinical evidence of a pregnancy. This is not a rare phenomenon, and, as noted in previous chapters, we do not feel that centers should include these biochemical pregnancies in their statistics indicating success.

CLINICAL PREGNANCY. In this case not only is there a positive pregnancy test, but we can also find other evidence of a pregnancy. The earliest evidence of a clinical pregnancy would consist of finding a pregnancy sac with or without fetal parts or a fetal heartbeat on an ultrasound examination. This is a very exciting moment for the couple, and we encourage the father to be present for this first ultrasound.

However, the pregnancy is subject to all the risks encountered by any pregnancy, including miscarriage and other conditions that can lead to a poor outcome. In addition, there has been a minor increase in premature labor in IVF pregnancies in addition to that resulting from multiple births.

LIVE BIRTH. This is the outcome we are all working toward. But even with the birth of a live baby, there can be the same chance of birth defects as there is in the general population. So the outcome we are hoping for is the birth of a healthy, normal baby.

You cannot assume that we will achieve this goal based only on a positive pregnancy test. Our joy at hearing that the pregnancy test is positive must be tempered with a small dose of caution. Placing too much emphasis on the positive pregnancy test can lead to great disappointment if it turns out to signify only a biochemical pregnancy or a clinical pregnancy that is later lost through miscarriage or other accident of pregnancy.

Theresa's reaction following a biochemical pregnancy is a good illustration of how deep the disappointment can be. She, happily, had a positive pregnancy test following her IVF cycle. Now, you must understand that positive pregnancy tests do evoke very strong emotions not only in the couple, but also among the IVF staff as well. Theresa was a very outgoing person and had become friendly with almost everyone on the staff. Thus, when her pregnancy test was positive, there was much crying and hugging and congratulations from the staff. Theresa interpeted this activity to mean that the baby was practically in her arms. When her positive test turned out to indicate only a biochemical pregnancy, her disappointment was especially intense. She felt that the positive response from the IVF staff made her disappointment more painful. Fortunately, several months following this disappointment she became pregnant as the result of a frozen embryo transfer and is currently doing well in her pregnancy. But because of this incident, we have instructed our staff, including physicians, to be mindful of the fact that the positive pregnancy test is news to be tempered with cautious optimism.

Consequently, these are the instructions we usually give to patients who have a positive pregnancy test:

1. We offer our congratulations, but modulate our joy with an admonition that although the positive test is good news, there is still a long way to go until they get to hold their baby. It's really too bad that we have to be somewhat pessimistic at this very happy news, but we feel it is our role to present all the facts to the couple in the proper perspective.

2. The woman should not engage in very heavy activity. That includes lifting, heavy housework, and exercise. Other than those precautions, she may engage in normal activity.

3. A daily prenatal vitamin is recommended. Until she sees her obstetrician for her first prenatal visit, any over-the-counter prenatal vitamin is adequate.

4. Intercourse with or without orgasm and other means of achieving orgasm can lead to uterine contractions that may interfere with the implanting embryo and therefore are not recommended until after the first twelve weeks. This extra-cautious approach started early in our own program several years ago, and, as a result or coincidentally, we experienced a very low rate of miscarriage. Understandably, we have continued to advise this precaution, and our rate of pregnancy loss has continued to be lower than the national average. Bleeding is common in ART pregnancies, probably due to multiple implantations. This may be the reason that the uterus is not quite as stable as in other pregnancies.

5. Progesterone will be continued, but now in the form of vaginal suppositories rather than injections. If there is any problem using the

suppositories or significant bleeding occurs, the injections are resumed. Some vaginal bleeding occurs in a large number of pregnancies, including IVF pregnancies, and does not necessarily mean that a miscarriage is occurring.

6. We recommend that the mother-to-be avoid caffeine, alcohol, smoking, and *all* drugs—including over-the-counter preparations and, of course, any recreational drugs. The only exception is acetaminophen (Tylenol, Datril, Anacin-3), which may be taken for aches and pains and should be taken to reduce fever.

7. She should return to the center for her first pregnancy ultrasound two weeks after the pregnancy test. At this time we will usually see the pregnancy sac or sacs, some evidence of fetal development and possibly fetal heart motion. We will know, with some degree of accuracy, how many pregnancies are present. The main reason for doing this scan is to alert us to the chance of a tubal pregnancy if we do not see a normally placed sac, with a fetus, in the uterus.

If the scan indicates a normal single pregnancy, twins, or triplets, we usually refer the patient on to her own obstetrician. The question of whether her own obstetrician is well equipped to take care of an IVF pregnancy is frequently asked by successful IVF patients. In general, we feel that any well-trained and experienced obstetrician is qualified to manage a single or twin IVF pregnancy. In the case of triplets, we would recommend discussing the resources available in her community to handle high-risk pregnancy. In the unlikely event of quadruplets or more, we feel that referral to a high-risk specialist is indicated.

IS THERE A GREATER CHANCE OF MISCARRIAGE?

As we indicated above when we cited the three possible outcomes from a positive pregnancy test, there is a significant risk of early loss of a clinical pregnancy through miscarriage. There is some variation among programs in their incidence of early pregnancy loss. The 1988 results from the National IVF/ET Registry from the American Fertility Society indicates an overall miscarriage rate of 24 percent and an ectopic pregnancy rate of 5 percent based on clinical pregnancies.

But if you look at pregnancies not conceived by ART procedures in women who are one week late, one large study documented a 22 percent rate of miscarriage. Just as with ART procedures, there is also a significant rate of biochemical pregnancy in "normal" couples trying to conceive. Therefore any increase in early pregnancy loss attributable to these procedures is very minor.

ARE IVF PREGNANCIES HIGH-RISK?

It is apparent that with multiple pregnancies involving three or more fetuses there is substantially more risk to the pregnancy than if there were just one or two fetuses present. Even the occurrence of twins increases the chance of obstetrical problems such as premature labor. But aside from the increased risk from multiple births, are IVF pregnancies in themselves at higher risk than those occurring naturally? Some studies have found a small but detectable increase in premature labor aside from that which occurs with multiple pregnancy. It is not clear whether this is related to the underlying infertility problem or to the ART procedure itself. But, according to a study of ninety-five IVF single pregnancies released from the University of Pennsylvania, IVF itself did not predispose the pregnancy to different
- length of gestation
- birth weight
- Apgar scores
- caesarean-section rate
- postdelivery blood count
- abnormal third-trimester bleeding
- infant or maternal survival
- incidence of medical or surgical complications of pregnancy
- premature labor
- rate of pregnancy-induced hypertension

MULTIPLE PREGNANCY

In the 1988 IVF data, the incidence of multiple deliveries was 19 percent of the clinical pregnancies, with 2.9 percent ending with the delivery of triplets or greater. In 1988 GIFT procedures, the rates were similar, with a total of 892 babies delivered, including 159 sets of twins (24 percent of clinical pregnancies) and thirty-four sets of triplets (5 percent of clinical pregnancies). The twin pregnancies can be managed fairly easily within most community resources, but it is the high-level multiple pregnancy that leads to concern about complications. In a recent review of twin pregnancies, preterm labor was observed in 58.8 percent of the cases, with 52 percent of the mothers delivering before thirty-six weeks. With triplets or more, the obstetrical outcome is significantly worse than in singleton or even twin pregnancies.

For the couple confronted by a multiple pregnancy with more than four fetuses (high-level multiple pregnancy), the options are few. To continue the pregnancy would lead to a very high chance of prematurity with its associated problems. With triplets or quadruplets, this is a realistic alternative. Although aborting some of the fetuses while leaving others to continue (selective termination) will directly harm some of the fetuses, it may offer the only hope of a successful outcome. An example of the danger of high-level multiple pregnancy is the highly publicized 1985 California septuplets case. Four of the babies died within one month of delivery and it is reported that all three survivors have cerebral palsy. Another possibility would be to avoid these serious potential consequences of prematurity by terminating the entire pregnancy. However, it would be a cruel irony for these patients who had tried for so long to conceive to then have to terminate a pregnancy because of a multiple gestation.

It is because of this dilemma facing couples with high-level multiple pregnancies that selective termination was developed. At first hearing, this idea sounds abhorrent. But when you realize that this may be the only way to save any of the fetuses, it becomes an option to consider. Actually, selective termination is considered appropriate in one of two circumstances. The first is fairly clear-cut. It can be used when one fetus in a set of twins has a serious birth defect or genetic abnormality. Less clear-cut is the situation that can occur as the result of infertility treatment, a multiple pregnancy of four or more fetuses. Most authorities agree, however, that it should not be used to reduce twins to a single pregnancy. In the case of triplets, in individual cases, it might be considered.

In skilled hands selective termination can be done with very little discomfort and with a low chance of disturbing the pregnancy. The most recent data show that following reduction of a high-level multiple pregnancy to twins, there is a 75 percent to 80 percent chance of producing live-born twins with an adequate amount of time in the uterus. As you would expect, the most common complication is miscarriage of the entire pregnancy. This is a relatively new procedure, but there are now doctors with sufficient experience for the chance of complications to be very low. One expert called selective termination "a lousy solution but the best hope for this problem." An international registry has been established to learn about the natural history of high-level multiple pregnancies and the operative statistics for selective termination.

As with most medical conditions, the best treatment is prevention. Although this problem cannot be prevented in all cases, proper monitoring of fertility drugs and limitation of numbers of eggs or embryos to be transferred will go a long way toward preventing high-level multiple pregnancy.

WILL MY BABY BE NORMAL?

One of the most frequent questions we hear regarding ART pregnancies is "Will my baby be normal?" The answer is that, as far we can determine, the incidence of birth defects is no different than in pregnancies conceived normally. This statement includes embryos that have been frozen. In the 1987 data from the National IVF Registry, among 1367 clinical pregnancies there were nine chromosomal abnormalities, all but one in women age thirty-four or greater. In addition, there were ten birth defects among these pregnancies for a rate actually slightly lower than the rate in the general population. The one exception to this blanket reassurance is a report from the Australia and New Zealand Perinatal Statistics Unit. Out of 1694 IVF and GIFT births there were thirty-seven major malformations (2.2 percent), which was not different from the expected percentage. However, six infants had spina bifida and four had a specific heart defect, more than expected. This finding has not been duplicated in the United States or Europe. Even if this slight increase was directly related to the ART procedures, it is very minor compared with the increase that occurs with age.

According to an August 1989 report in *The New York Times*, a study of eighty-three children born as the result of in vitro fertilization showed them to be as healthy and mentally alert as a group of children born through natural conception.

Despite this encouraging news, we urge women with ART pregnancies to take advantage of all the diagnostic tests that are appropriate and available for them. Women over thirty-four are encouraged to consider amniocentesis or chromosomal evaluation of the pregnancy. Those having amniocentesis can check for open defects of the tissue covering the brain and spinal cord (neural tube defects) by checking the alphafetoprotein levels in the amniotic fluid. Alphafetoprotein blood screening is widely available to those not having amniocentesis to check for neural tube defects and, in addition, chromosomal and other abnormalities. In view of the one report regarding spina bifida, we recommend this test be done routinely and, if amniocentesis is not done, a thorough eighteen-week ultrasound examination may be suggested (some argue that this should be done in every pregnancy anyway). We generally do not recommend chorionic villus sampling to detect chromosomal defects because it has a slightly higher risk of miscarriage, a situation we especially want to avoid in a woman who has only been able to conceive by means of an ART procedure.

FINDING AN OBSTETRICIAN

Since you have probably spent years in your quest for this pregnancy, it is very likely that you already know a general obstetrician and gynecologist. Assuming that you like and have confidence in him or her and that you have a single or twin pregnancy, you have no more looking to do. A well-trained obstetrician is experienced in dealing with such cases.

If you do not have your own physician who can take care of your pregnancy, you can use most of the criteria you have found in Chapter 8 to make a list of physicians who may become your new Dr. Perfect, the obstetrician. It is most likely that the physicians who participated in your ART procedure do not deliver babies, although there are exceptions. However, your fertility doctor will likely be a good resource to obtain a referral to an obstetrician. In fact, he or she naturally wants to be sure you receive good care.

There are some specific considerations in choosing a doctor to deliver your baby that differ from those in selecting a fertility specialist. First of all, many obstetricians will offer a free consultation for you to become acquainted before you sign on the dotted line. This is an opportunity for you to become familiar with the doctor's philosophy and demeanor. There are many choices to be made with regard to your obstetrical care, not only relating to the mechanics of delivery but also in the selection of prenatal testing, location of hospital for delivery, method of analgesia and anesthesia, and availability of consultation in case of complications, to name a few. You will want to make sure that the physician who will guide you through this pregnancy starts with the same basic philosophy you do.

When you do get to meet with the physician, you should plan to get as much information as you can in a period of five to ten minutes. We suggest you focus your limited time on three areas which will give you a pretty good idea of his or her philosophy:

- Availability
- Substitute coverage
- Flexibility

1. How available are you to answer my questions?

The ideal answer would be total availability—a patient's dream, but in reality an impossibility. Even a doctor has a private life, with its duties and crises and even some time off for good behavior. What you are trying to establish here is to what extent your calls for information will be fielded by the doctor. Or will you be speaking to the nurse and not have access to the doctor except in medical emergencies. Some women prefer discussing most things with the nurse; others prefer the physician. It's wise to obtain the office policy on that in advance as it may avoid potential hassles and feelings of neglect later on.

2. How available are you for deliveries? When you're not available, who covers for you?

Needless to say, this is an extremely important issue. Usually you will be told that he or she has a regular coverage arrangement with physicians who follow the same general philosophy and that your care will be the same no matter which physician happens to be on call. Unfortunately, some physicians who regularly deliver babies do not have formalized coverage arrangements with other equally qualified physicians. When they do, often it's with a friend or acquaintance who may not share the doctor's or (more important) your philosophy. For example, there can be differences in the use of pain medications during labor, the types of anesthetics, and different views as to the need for caesarean deliveries.

In answer to this question you want to hear that there *is* a coverage policy and that you have the option to meet one or all of the doctors who provide this service. You should flinch if the doctor says "Don't worry... I'll be there." Too many women have been burned by this insincere promise. We know of one woman, a lawyer, who was carrying twins and kept asking her physician who would be there if he was unable to attend the delivery. He kept insisting that he delivered all of his own patients. Well, you guessed it! When she had an emergency necessitating the delivery of the twins, he was nowhere to be found and she had to rely on the luck of the draw. A physician who happened to be in the hospital responded and fortunately all turned out well. Remember, when it comes to delivering babies, the selection of a doctor is often only as good as his or her coverage.

3. What are your routine procedures for patients in labor?

Actually, no procedures are routine in labor. You don't want to hear the doctor rattle off a list of routines pertaining to enema, shave, IV, and other predelivery procedures. What you want to hear is that the doctor applies a degree of flexibility in dealing with patients in labor, that the patient's individual needs are an important consideration. You may be told that the hospital calls for specific routines during labor. Don't believe it. Chances are this doctor is hiding behind "hospital rules" in order to apply his or her own preferences. Inflexibility is not what you're looking for in a physician, despite the best credentials.

Those are the three big questions. The doctor's answers and any discussion surrounding them will, in all likelihood, consume the bulk of your allotted time, but should the meeting continue and the doctor has more time to answer questions, here are some more worthwhile ones.

4. How often do you perform a caesarean section?

The question can also be phrased "What is your C-section rate?" You're looking for a straightforward answer, for example "My C-section rate is 14 percent, which is consistent with what we do in the community" or "My rate is a little higher because I see many patients who are at high risk for complications, patients with diabetes, for example." An acceptable rule of thumb is a primary C-section rate (not including repeat caesareans) between 14 and 18 percent.

5. What are the reasons you induce labor? How often do you induce?

This issue refers to the use of drugs (Pitocin) to trigger the onset of labor. You'd like to hear the doctor say "I seldom do elective inductions. But I do induce occasionally for medical reasons such as diabetes, high blood pressure, premature rupture of the membranes, or when someone goes too far past her due date." If the doctor says "I like to induce everybody, it's much more convenient," that's not what you want to hear. It's a very questionable routine practice.

6. What is your fee?

The answer to this question is readily available at the front office. If you're comparison shopping, it might be wise to conduct a small survey in the community. Check with several offices and establish a range of fees. We do not recommend that you select a physician primarily on the basis of the lowest or highest fee. Just make sure that the fees you are being charged are within the range in your community.

The subject of fees raises the issue of medical insurance coverage, an issue that could determine if you have any choice of physician at all. In this era of prepaid health plans and preferred provider arrangements, your choice may be severely limited to those health professionals who are affiliated with the plan. If you belong to a health maintenance organization (HMO), this will certainly be the case. If you are under a preferred provider organization (PPO) plan, you stand to lose a portion of your insurance reimbursement if you see a physician who is not affiliated with your PPO. Unfortunately, many women discover too late that they're locked into the physician-access system that falls within their husbands' health insurance package from work, the two- or three-year-old plan he may have forgotten to tell his wife about.

While many physicians in these HMO and PPO plans are dedicated to practice quality medicine, they may differ with each other in regard to the management of obstetric patients. It may be difficult to ensure that all your needs are being met under these conditions and you may have to lobby strongly for what you want. For example, many HMOs have rules that you cannot see a physician until you are a certain number of weeks pregnant. As an IVF- or GIFT-pregnant patient, the early part of pregnancy is crucial and we feel you should be under a doctor's care at this time. You may, in some situations, have to fight for that right.

A WORD OF ADVICE

There is something amazing about pregnancy. You quickly become a believer in the old saying "One gives nothing so freely as advice" and begin to understand that free advice is worth what you have paid for it. You'll wonder if the news that someone is pregnant has the effect of triggering the advice-giving gene in people. Sometimes it will be difficult to separate wisdom from ignorance, fact from myth. You can count on being told that you must eat for two. Perhaps someone will caution you against raising your arms over your head since it might cause the umbilical cord to wrap itself around the baby's neck. At least one thoughtless individual will probably tell you that you should not be having a baby through IVF or GIFT because it's unnatural or that they are opposed to people having GIFT triplets because humans were not meant to have litters. You will also find that almost everyone who has had a baby wants to regale you with the gory details of her terrible three days in labor.

We recommend that the last piece of advice you take seriously from anyone other than your own health professionals is this: Don't take any advice from anyone other than your own health professionals. Either listen politely and forget it or tell the advice-giver that you are really not interested in what happened to his or her Aunt Tillie. If you have questions or concerns, ask your doctor, read or speak to your childbirth instructors, but don't take the advice of well-meaning friends or relatives.

GOOD LUCK!

You are about to embark upon one of the most exciting adventures of your life. We encourage you to learn as much as you can about pregnancy and the birth process through reading and classes so you can help make many of the choices which will confront you through this pregnancy. Good luck!

eleven

Donors

In this book we have described the latest techniques used to treat a variety of conditions that result in infertility. However, even sophisticated 1990s medical technology has limitations. When the best science has to offer is not enough, we are often forced to rely upon the replacement of faulty organs with donor organs, as when kidney failure requires a kidney transplant or end-stage cardiovascular disease requires a heart or lung transplant from a donor. In many of these cases the donor organ is donated after death, although for some a sibling or parent can provide an organ.

Donations of semen or eggs for the treatment of infertility are different. They are more akin to blood donations. There is so much reserve built into the human reproductive system that egg donors (and even more sperm donors) can donate their gametes on many occasions with essentially no significant depletion of their reserves. Sperm donation can be done every few days without any adverse effects on the donor. Egg donation cannot be done so often, but eggs certainly can be donated on more than one occasion.

We are at the point of being able to offer replacement of both male and female gametes when modern technology alone cannot repair or replace abnormalities in the male and female genital tract. There are four categories of donation in the treatment of infertility:

1. Sperm donation

2. Egg donation
3. Surrogate parenting—where the use of the uterus with or without eggs is donated
4. Adoption

Our discussion will center around the first two categories, since they are the ones most closely associated with ART procedures. Surrogate parenting is another topic in itself with many legal and ethical ramifications and has been thoroughly explored in other publications. Adoption is also a topic beyond the scope of this book. (References regarding surrogate parenting and adoption will be found in Appendix 2.)

SEMEN DONATION

The donation of semen for artificial insemination has been practiced for over a century. However, concerns during the last decade about complications related to the transmission of infectious diseases have resulted in changes in the practice of donor artificial insemination. These concerns resulted in the American Fertility Society issuing in February 1988 new guidelines for the use of donor insemination. Most of the changes in the guidelines relate to measures to try to avoid the transmission of sexually transmitted diseases, most notably AIDS.

Reasons for semen donation

The major indications for donor insemination are:
- The husband is irreversibly sterile from any cause.
- The husband has had a vasectomy and does not want to have it reversed.
- The husband has a low or marginal sperm count, antisperm antibodies, or some other condition where the male factor is thought to be the predominant cause of the infertility and cannot be overcome by other means.
- The husband has or is a carrier of a known hereditary disease.
- The husband has a problem with ejaculation that cannot be overcome by current technology.
- The wife is Rh-negative and severely sensitized to Rh-positive blood and the husband is Rh-positive.
- In ART procedures for all the above reasons and also in cases of

failure of fertilization in couples with a male factor or unexplained
infertility.

Making the decision

The decision to utilize donor insemination is at times difficult, but
many couples enter this treatment in a very matter-of-fact fashion.

Consider the case of Lorraine, twenty-four, and Steve, thirty-two.
Several years ago Steve was treated for testicular cancer with chemotherapy, which left his sperm count very low and most of those left
apparently damaged. Steve was told by his doctors, at the time he
received his chemotherapy, that he would never be able to have his
own children. When they had been married for two years and decided
to start a family, they came in requesting donor insemination with no
hesitation whatsoever. After being fully informed about the procedure
and about the selection of donors through a regional sperm bank, they
quickly signed the consents and went off to the cryobank to choose
their donor. It was important to them that the donor have as many
physical characteristics in common with Steve as possible.

When they returned for the first insemination based on Lorraine's
positive Ovustick, they proudly announced that they had chosen
"number 43." He had the same ethnic origin, hair and eye color,
general build, and educational background as Steve. Lorraine became
pregnant with her first insemination. They had a baby boy and were
so delighted with their son that they called the cryobank and placed
some of number 43's semen on reserve so that all of their children
would resemble one another. One year after the birth of their first son
they decided to have another baby. This time it took two tries before
Lorraine became pregnant, but they had another son. Again they kept
some of number 43's semen on reserve. We have just learned that they
have decided not to have any more children and have notified the
sperm bank that they would release the remaining specimens. They are
delighted with their two sons and are thankful to number 43.

But the decision for other couples to resort to donor insemination is
not so easy. Perhaps it was easier for Lorraine and Steve because Steve
had been prepared by his doctors when he underwent chemotherapy.
Sometimes the news that the man is infertile has such intense
emotional consequences that he is unable to accept the thought of
donor insemination. At other times a couple may be so concerned

about the genetic and medical histories of the donors and the potential spread of disease that they are unable to accept donor insemination despite assurances that proper screening and testing have been done. Cultural and religious influences often come into play. The couple considering the use of a donor must be fully informed about all aspects of the process and their consequences. They then must sign an informed consent statement including, depending on individual state laws, many or all of the following:

- The husband is treated in law as if he were the natural father of the child (twenty-nine states) and all children born shall be legitimate children and heirs to the couple's estate.
- They will never seek to identify the donor.
- There is no guarantee that insemination will result in a pregnancy.
- A certain percentage of children are born with physical or mental defects, and the occurrence of such defects is beyond the control of physicians.
- There is a very small risk of infection.
- Any pregnancy carries with it the risk of obstetrical complications or miscarriage.
- Semen from the same donor may not be available for all inseminations.
- Frozen sperm will be used.

Guidelines for semen donation

Once the couple has decided to utilize donor insemination, the process of selecting a sperm bank is the next step in the process. Since there are no objective criteria available to the lay public regarding the operation of sperm banks, the couple will have to rely on the advice of their physician in selecting one. However, there are some universally accepted principles and some of the right questions will let you know if the bank is following accepted guidelines.

1. Is the bank either adhering to screening standards established by the American Association of Tissue Banks (AATB) and/or do they follow the guidelines for the selection and screening of donors issued by the American Fertility Society (AFS)?

The answer should be yes. According to the standards of the AATB, the donor should be screened by two physicians for fertility, health, intelligence, and the absence of infectious disease, including AIDS screening. The minimal AFS screen includes insuring the absence in the donor and his close relatives of any nontrivial malformation, genetic disorder, familial disease, recessive genes for any disease, or chromosomal abnormalities. In addition, he must be free of psychosis, epilepsy, juvenile diabetes, and early coronary disease.

2. How do you screen for AIDS?

The AFS guidelines excludes as donors any men who have engaged in any of the known high-risk behaviors related to the spread of AIDS. In addition, AIDS antibody tests should be done periodically and the semen should be quarantined until a follow-up AIDS antibody test, done six months after the specimen is provided, is found to be negative for the AIDS antibody.

3. Do you use fresh specimens?

According to the latest revision of the guidelines published in February 1988, it is the position of the AFS that the use of fresh semen for donor insemination is no longer warranted. Although there may be some decrease in pregnancy rates and/or increase in the length of time to conceive utilizing frozen (cryopreserved) semen, it is the only way to provide maximum safety against the transmission of AIDS. In addition, the AATB, U.S. Food and Drug Administration, and the Centers for Disease Control all recommend the exclusive use of frozen semen for donation.

4. Isn't frozen semen less effective than fresh?

It is thought that with conventional artificial insemination the overall pregnancy rate when frozen specimens are utilized for donor insemination appears to be less than with fresh semen and the duration of therapy is therefore prolonged. For example, a recent study from the University of Kansas comparing characteristics of frozen and fresh donor semen found a marked reduction in all aspects of semen quality in the frozen specimens. However, there was no significant difference in cumulative pregnancy rates and they concluded that if minimum criteria for ejaculate quality is met, cryopreserved ejaculates can provide an effective and safe alternative to the use of fresh semen. With ART procedures, there is no reduction in success with frozen sperm.

But even if there were a lower pregnancy rate, frozen semen provides several distinct advantages that more than make up for the slightly reduced efficacy. The use of frozen semen reduces the risk of acquiring a sexually transmitted disease by allowing more time for screening as well as providing a quarantine period for diseases such as AIDS and hepatitis-B. It allows greater flexibility in scheduling inseminations and donor selection. The frozen specimen is available at any time while the donor himself may not be. Finally, it allows one specimen to be divided into several doses, which is very economical. Although the processing and storage adds somewhat to the cost, it is more than made up by the advantages.

5. Besides AIDS, what other diseases do you screen for?

The AFS recommends exclusion of a donor if he has had more than one sexual partner or symptoms of a sexually transmitted disease within six months or a past history at any time of warts, herpes, chronic hepatitis, or exclusion as a blood donor unless for a noninfectious reason. In donors continuing to participate in the program, they recommend a physical examination and testing every six months for:

- gonorrhea
- chlamydia
- trichomonas
- hepatitis-B
- syphilis
- AIDS

According to an Office of Technology Assessment report, "Artificial Insemination: practice in the United States," during a twelve-month period during 1986 and 1987, 11,000 physicians performed artificial inseminations with husband's or donor semen on 172,000 women in the United States. They estimate that 30,000 births occurred as the result of the donor inseminations performed during that year. These numbers suggest a five- to eight-fold increase in donor insemination pregnancies compared to a period studied eight years previously.

Despite all of the above recommendations, the 1987 survey showed that 22 percent of the 11,000 physicians performing donor insemination used fresh semen exclusively. Less than half of the physicians using fresh semen screened for AIDS and only about one-quarter of them tested for other sexually transmitted diseases. Less than half performed any genetic screening on donors.

This has resulted in a call for legislation in various states and in Congress to require medical and genetic screening of donors and even to set up a national data bank for semen donors to maintain their medical and genetic histories and make them available to the recipient.

How it is done

When dealing with the couple having only a male factor problem in conventional infertility treatment, the donor sperm can be placed in an insemination cup that is then positioned against the cervix and left there for several hours. Some physicians inject a small amount into the cervical mucus before placing the remainder in the cup against the cervix. In the absence of other factors, this method will be adequate. We recommend the timing of the insemination be done by means of the LH-surge kit to help insure accuracy and to allow use of only one insemination, which is more convenient and cost-effective for the patient.

If, in addition to a male factor problem there is a cervical factor or stimulation of ovulation with clomiphene where the cervical mucus may be deficient, the frozen donor specimen can be washed with a special medium and intrauterine insemination can be performed. Some centers now are washing all donor specimens and then inseminating them directly into the uterus. In a recent publication, doctors reported a monthly conception rate of 24 percent with an ongoing pregnancy rate of 18 percent using intrauterine insemination using specimens containing a minimum of 24 million cryopreserved motile sperm.

When donor semen is used in ART procedures, it is prepared in a manner similar to fresh specimens to be used to inseminate the eggs in the laboratory in IVF, ZIFT, PROST, and TE(S)T. With GIFT procedures, the prepared semen is mixed with the eggs to be placed in the fallopian tube.

Costs

The use of cryopreserved donor semen does not significantly increase the costs of conventional infertility treatment or ART procedures. As of January 1989, the cost of a single frozen specimen from a well-known sperm bank in Los Angeles was under $100. When a number of specimens were ordered, the cost per specimen was modestly reduced. The cost of the insemination process, without washing the sperm, would be between $50 and $100. If the physician washes the specimen and places it in the uterus, the cost would be approximately $100 for the wash and insemination.

EGG DONATION

While the donation of semen has been practiced for more than a century, the history of egg donation spans only a few years. Its development has paralleled others in assisted reproductive technology as it became understood that there are a group of women who, for any number of basic reasons, were unable to reproduce because of lack of eggs (oocytes) or development of poor-quality eggs that either do not fertilize or fertilize poorly or result in consistently poor-quality embryos.

Reasons for egg donation

Prime candidates for utilizing donor eggs are patients in the following circumstances:

- The wife has amenorrhea or anovulation that has not responded to fertility medications.
- The wife has laboratory evidence of premature ovarian failure, usually manifested in elevated gonadotropin levels (FSH and LH).
- The wife has demonstrated poor follicle development with stimulation due to pelvic adhesions, a paucity of ovarian tissue because of previous surgery, or for unknown reasons.
- The wife carries a genetic disease or chromosomal defect likely to be passed on to her offspring, resulting in miscarriage or an abnormal baby.
- The couple may have had multiple failed ART procedures, particularly with poor egg quality being found.
- The wife may be over forty and may choose egg donation because of a dramatically higher rate of success.

Making the decision

The decision to utilize donor eggs can be made in two circumstances. It seems to be an easier decision to make if the patient has a sister or friend who wishes to donate eggs for her. When the donor is unknown, the decision is similar to the decision to use donor semen.

Karen, thirty-two, had a long history of endometriosis, including two operations resulting in the removal of one ovary and about half of the other. After many years of attempting to become pregnant without success, she decided to enter the IVF program. She produced six eggs with her first attempt. Four fertilized and were transferred, but she did not get pregnant. In her second attempt, she had only three eggs, all of which fertilized, but without success. With subsequent cycles, she stimulated poorly. It was felt that pelvic adhesions and lack of ovarian substance was impairing her ability to produce an adequate response to the stimulating hormones. The possibility of using an egg donor was discussed with both Karen and her husband, and she suggested that her sister might be willing to donate. Her sister was thirty-four and already had two children, but Karen thought that her sister might not want to do it and was a little reluctant to ask. As it turned out, her sister immediately agreed and said that she had been thinking of offering to donate before she was asked. In fact, it has been our experience that sisters of infertile women are usually more than happy to provide this service. Karen is currently pregnant as the result of her sister's donated eggs.

As with the recipients of donor semen, the recipients of donor eggs must be fully informed of every aspect of the procedure, including all potential risks, and must sign an informed consent outlining the following:

- The anonymous donor will not know the identity of the husband and wife and the husband and wife will not know the identity of the donor.
- The anonymous donor's information is supplied by the donor, so there are limitations to the accuracy of this information. Even though laboratory tests are performed on the donor, the transmission of infection is still possible.
- The recipient is responsible for the medical costs of screening and stimulating the donor and harvesting the eggs as well as financial compensation for the efforts, time, and inconvenience of an anonymous donor.
- From the moment of conception, the husband and wife will accept the child as their own legitimate child or children and heirs.
- There is no guarantee that a normal pregnancy will occur.
- The husband and wife understand that a certain percentage of babies are born with defects and that this is beyond the control of the doctors.

Guidelines for egg donation

As already indicated, donors fall into one of two categories: the relative or friend who agrees to donate and the anonymous donor. Incidentally, the friends and relatives are screened with the same intensity as are the anonymous donors because friends and relatives can have significant histories of genetic problems and can also carry sexually transmitted diseases. Since there are no established guidelines for the selection and screening of egg donors, we have adopted the basic principles used in the AFS guidelines for semen donors. We suggest that you check on the guidelines for selection and screening of the program you are considering. If you are planning to use an egg donor, that prospective donor must:

- Have no congenital malformations in herself or close relatives
- Have no genetic disorder in herself or her family
- Have no familial disease with a genetic component such as juvenile diabetes
- Not be or have a sex partner in an AIDS risk group
- Not be an IV drug user
- Not have a past history of genital herpes, genital warts, chronic hepatitis, or have been excluded from giving blood other than for a noninfectious reason
- Be under age thirty-five

If the prospective donor passes this historical scrutiny, she will be subjected to a physical examination and testing to rule out the possibility of congenital anomalies, chronic illness, or sexually transmitted disease. Blood tests will be obtained for hepatitis-B, syphilis, and AIDS. She must be in a monogamous relationship and her partner must agree to be tested for AIDS.

Because of a scarcity of egg donors compared to semen donors, the characteristics used to match a donor to a recipient are usually limited to ethnicity, hair and eye color, and, in some cases, education. The recipient couple can ask for any set of criteria, but the stricter their criteria, the less the chance that they will find a suitable donor; most couples are accepting our two major criteria.

The major difference between semen and egg donation is that the egg donor does accept some risk to herself in the process. First, she has to undergo significant stimulation of the ovaries to produce the number of eggs necessary to make the donation meaningful and cost-effective. Secondly, the retrieval method by vaginal ultrasound or laparoscopy does carry with it some risk.

There are two categories of women who donate eggs anonymously. In the first category is the woman who is planning to have a laparoscopy to have her tubes tied and decides that she would like to donate eggs to an infertile couple. In the second is the woman who has decided to donate her eggs for altruistic reasons without having the need for any operation. For women in the first category, the risk is easily justified because they are planning to undergo the risk of laparoscopy anyway and the additional risk of the stimulation is small. However, reports have indicated that it is difficult to recruit women in this category. The most frequent reason for declining to participate in conjunction with a tubal ligation is the perception that if a pregnancy were to result, the child would be partly theirs. It has been the experience of many centers that it is easier to find women in the second category who are willing to accept the risk because donating eggs to an infertile couple meets some need of theirs. These women probably represent a philosophically select group, emotionally committed to the idea regardless of the inconvenience and possible risk. They are akin to the large number of people we hear about who come forth to donate a kidney to a complete stranger or the thousands who offer to be tested as bone marrow donors for a young cancer victim. There are people who meet some of their own needs by helping others in this way.

In view of the inconvenience and, more crucial, the potential risk, the donors are thoroughly informed about the procedure and must sign a consent form that includes these points:

- She will have to undergo tests for sexually transmitted diseases, including AIDS.
- She must verify that she has not had contact with a person with AIDS, used intravenous drugs, or had a sexual partner who, to her knowledge, has ever had a sexual contact with a homosexual male, IV drug user, or someone with AIDS.
- She agrees not to have sexual intercourse from the start of her menstrual period and during medication.
- She agrees to take fertility drugs to obtain multiple eggs for donation.

- The risks of the fertility drugs and the retrieval procedure are listed.
- She relinquishes any claim to or jurisdiction over offspring that might result from the use of her eggs in the recipient.

The donors do receive compensation for their time away from work or their families and for their inconvenience. In selecting an amount for this honorarium, we want to give the donor something large enough to compensate her adequately for her services, yet we did not want to make it so high that it would encourage women to donate eggs in order to make money. We settled on an honorarium of $1000 for anonymous donors, both for those who are having their tubes tied and those who do not need surgery and are donating for purely altruistic reasons.

A bond of sorts is established between the anonymous donor and recipient although they never meet. The donors are frequently concerned about the results and call to find out the outcome of the pregnancy test. They tell us to wish the recipient luck and often ask us to "give her a hug for me." On occasion the recipient will give something to the donor. One donor's egg pickup was scheduled for Valentine's Day and the recipient bought her a gold heart-shaped locket with a ruby surrounded by little diamonds. That recipient had twins. The recipients tell us to "tell her thanks" and to indicate how grateful they are. Perhaps IVF using donor eggs would be better called "GIFT."

From our available pool of donors, we attempt to make the best match primarily by ethnicity and hair and eye color. When there are other specific requests, we try to match them, but the pool of egg donors is much more limited than semen donors. Once the donor has been selected by the couple and is ready to start, the process begins.

How it is done

Since the use of an egg donor is actually part of the IVF program, the same basic steps are required, although with some modifications:
1. Ripening of the eggs in the donor while the recipient is being primed.
2. Retrieval of the eggs from the donor.
3. Fertilization of the eggs with the husband's sperm and growth of the resulting embryos in the laboratory.
4. Transfer of the embryos into the uterus of the recipient.

Egg development

The process is very similar to that of an IVF procedure. The donor is seen about one week following an ovulation which has been documented by a urinary ovulation detector or BBT rise. She comes in for an initial vaginal ultrasound scan to evaluate the baseline appearance of her pelvic organs and a urine test to prove ovulation has occurred. If the scan is normal and the test shows evidence that ovulation has occurred, she is started on daily injections of Lupron. These injections can be given by her husband or self-administered. After 12 days of Lupron, or later if her menstrual period has not started, she returns for another scan and a blood test to see if her estrogen level is suppressed. A normal scan and a suppressed estrogen level will allow us to start her on hMG injections. The injections are usually given by a standard protocol based on her weight since it is likely that she has had no previous experience with hMG. These injections are more difficult to give since they are a larger volume and are given deep in the muscle. It is rare that a person can self-administer this shot, and the husband or a friend is generally taught how to do this.

On the sixth day of hMG, the donor returns for a scan which may result in a modification of her dosage. Repeat scans are done every one to three days. When the follicles reach close to mature size, daily blood tests for estrogen and progesterone are done. When the size and number of the follicles and resulting estrogen level indicate that they are mature, HCG is given and preparations are made to retrieve the eggs.

Meanwhile, the recipient is being prepared for the process. If she is still menstruating, she will have been placed on Lupron to totally suppress her own cycle and will be maintained on the Lupron until her donor is ready.

When the donor is on her sixth day of Lupron, the recipient will be started on estrogen by means of the estradiol skin patch (Estraderm) which will be increased in number every few days to simulate a normal cycle. As the eggs reach maturity and the donor receives the HCG, the recipient will be started on progesterone injections to prime her endometrium to receive the embryos.

A typical cycle when the recipient is still ovulating would look like this:

	RECIPIENT	DONOR
Six days after ovulation	Lupron	Lupron
Day 6 of Lupron (donor)	Estraderm	Lupron
Day 12 of Lupron (donor)	Estraderm	Lupron/hMG
When eggs are mature	Estraderm	HCG
Day after HCG	Estraderm	Pre-retrieval
	Progesterone	visit
2 days after HCG	Estraderm	Retrieval
	Progesterone	
2 days after Retrieval	Embryo Transfer	—
	Estraderm	
	Progesterone	

Egg retrieval

The egg retrieval procedure in the donor who does not need a laparoscopy for tubal ligation will be identical to the patient undergoing vaginal ultrasound egg retrieval for IVF. If the donor is one who is planning a tubal ligation, the egg retrieval by laparoscopy will be similar to egg retrieval performed in the patient with an IVF laparoscopic retrieval or the retrieval portion of a GIFT procedure. A very recent study has indicated that it is possible to retrieve oocytes without stimulation of the ovaries, by maturing them in follicular fluid from mature follicles from other stimulated cycles. In one reported case five embryos were transferred to an egg donor recipient, who delivered healthy triplets. As an extra precaution we give a week of antibiotics to make the chance of infection as remote as possible.

Fertilization

The eggs are taken to the laboratory and incubated for a period of time before insemination. The husband of the recipient will deposit a semen specimen in a sterile container by masturbation. The insemination technique and observation of the embryos will be no different from the average IVF cycle.

Embryo transfer or replacement

The embryos which were, forty-eight or so hours ago, eggs obtained from the donor are now prepared to be transferred into the uterus of the recipient. Again, the transfer will be conducted in exactly the same manner as the transfer in any other IVF cycle.

Costs

The cost of an IVF cycle employing donor eggs would be the same as for any other IVF cycle, but with the addition of the honorarium for the donor ($1000 in our program) as well as the costs of advertising, recruitment, and screening the donors and testing for infections (about $1000). All the costs relating to stimulation of the ovaries and retrieval of the eggs would be the same as with the regular IVF patient except that they are performed on the donor but paid for by the recipient couple. In fact, the cost of stimulation might be somewhat less in the donor than in an infertile IVF patient since a fertile woman might require less stimulation. Then, finally, there are expenses related to suppressing and replacing the recipient's menstrual cycle and the hormonal replacement and monitoring of the early pregnancy. If the cycle is successful, these would be an additional $1000.

Success and failure

In the 1988 experience reported by the National IVF-ET Registry of the American Fertility Society, twenty-six of the clinics reporting performed IVF with donated eggs. One hundred thirty patients underwent a total of 158 donor transfers. Fifty-one (32 percent) of the transfers resulted in a clinical pregnancy. The fifty-one pregnancies resulted in thirty-six live births (23 percent) with twelve sets of twins and one set of triplets. Since the time of that report many more donor cycles have been done. Just as with the 1988 report, the rate of ongoing pregnancy is substantially higher than with routine IVF. In our own experience, we have completed eighteen egg-donation cycles in which fertilization was successful with eleven pregnancies of which nine are ongoing (one triplet, three twins, and five singletons) beyond twelve weeks. In three other cases prior fertilization failure had been attributed to poor eggs but again occurred with normal donor eggs.

The level of persistence of patients who succeed through gamete donation is remarkable. Marcy, in her late thirties, had three ectopic pregnancies, but by the time IVF was attempted she failed to stimulate and was found to be approaching menopause. Her sister offered to donate eggs; on the second attempt with her sister's eggs, she became pregnant and delivered triplets. At the annual Father's Day celebration at the IVF Center, Marcy's husband gave thanks for their success and attributed their triplets to the fact that they went through the anguish of losing three babies to ectopic pregnancies.

Sometimes the margin between success and failure is very small. Carolyn, in her early forties, had only a sliver of an ovary left after repeated surgeries. Her cousin offered to donate. However, the cousin's ovaries were unusually difficult to reach and only two eggs were obtained. Of those, only one fertilized. The transfer of that sole embryo resulted in a healthy pregnancy. Talk about "little miracles"!

SURROGATE PARENTING AND ADOPTION

These two subjects are beyond the scope of this book and have been dealt with extensively in books on those subjects alone. Consult Appendix 2 for resource recommendations on these subjects. The only aspect of surrogacy we will mention here is surrogate IVF.

SURROGATE IVF

If a woman's ovaries are functioning but she has had her uterus removed or it is abnormal, it is possible to retrieve her eggs, fertilize them with her husband's sperm, and transfer them to a surrogate who then carries the pregnancy. Several pregnancies have been achieved, including the well-known story of a woman in her forties who carried a pregnancy for her daughter. This procedure allows the infertile couple to have their own genetic offspring. It also has the potential for a higher pregnancy rate because the embryos can be transferred to a normal unstimulated recipient. Since the pregnancy is genetically unrelated to the surrogate, the potential for emotional attachment and consequent legal entanglements is reduced. Also, because the child is solely the genetic offspring of the infertile couple, the chance for any legal ruling assigning a parental right to the surrogate should be small.

Unfortunately, any form of reproduction involving a surrogate is very involved and expensive. Surrogates must be carefully screened and the legal documents must be thoroughly and skillfully prepared. It is probably best for a small number of programs to provide this service because of the organizational aspects required.

BEYOND DONORS

The use of donor eggs is just one of the more exciting new aspects. of assisted reproduction that is already producing results in the form of live births. As this young technology moves well into its second decade, we will guide you through the areas where we see the most promise for progress in the next twelve years of ART in Chapter 12.

twelve

The Future
Looks Bright

I wish they could all get their children; that's not going to happen. We will be able, in the next seven to eight years, to double our success rate. I know that we can.

Gary Hodgen, Ph.D.,
Scientific Director, Jones Institute
on *48 Hours* (CBS News),
September 1989

THE FUTURE AND ASSISTED REPRODUCTIVE TECHNOLOGY

The first dozen years of IVF have seen tremendous progress—from a time when teams of researchers worked for years to achieve just one success to today, when some skilled and experienced teams can achieve a term pregnancy in one fifth to one quarter of egg retrievals. During this period problems with stimulation have been reduced, with cancellation of a treatment cycle becoming an uncommon event. Egg retrieval has been vastly simplified by the development of ultrasound-guided follicle aspiration under local anesthesia. Finally, with embryo freezing, a further pregnancy can be achieved without the risk or cost of another stimulation and egg retrieval. Can we expect as much progress in the next dozen years? Probably not, but there are going to be continued breakthroughs.

Uniformity of results

First of all, to say that only some teams achieve good success is not enough. All patients can't be treated by these few centers. One challenge for the next few years is to make results more consistent so that all teams are realizing good results. Since there is currently little agreement over which techniques are preferable, this sort of uniformity can only be achieved by the less successful clinics adopting techniques used by highly successful programs. We would argue that this is precisely what is necessary to bring the less successful programs up to par.

Financial resources

Besides having IVF in a highly successful program, the next most important factor influencing the chance of success is the number of cycles a couple goes through. Here the problem of lack of insurance coverage is the major impediment to success. Given adequate financial support, the procedure is now simple enough to allow couples to tolerate going through four attempts. At our current rate of 26 percent term pregnancy rate per retrieval, a woman under age forty would reach a cumulative rate of 70 percent at the conclusion of four attempts. Add to that frozen embryo pregnancies and the rate would be at least 75 to 80 percent, taking into account recent improvements in freezing results.

Laboratory techniques

Laboratory techniques will improve, resulting in progressively less of a difference in the chance of pregnancy between IVF, which depends entirely on laboratory quality, and GIFT, which substitutes the fallopian tube environment for the laboratory. As techniques continue to improve for producing pregnancy in women with open tubes without having to resort to ART techniques, it seems inevitable to us that GIFT will play less and less of a role in the future. One example of this is the increased viability of embryos grown on a "helper" layer of animal fetal cells.

Uterine receptivity

Clearly, the endometrium in a stimulated cycle is less receptive than in the normal cycle. Also, the uterine cavity may not be as supportive at the time of embryo transfer two days after retrieval as it normally is at three to four days after ovulation—when the embryo normally moves from the tube to the uterus. This effect is most obvious with the doubling of the ongoing pregnancy rate that occurs with egg donation in which embryos are placed into a normal endometrial cavity that has been exposed to progesterone for about seventy-two hours. With greater understanding of the effect of the state of the endometrium, modifications in the hormonal balance in the early luteal phase could dramatically increase successful implantation. Such improvements together with better transfer technique could obviate the need for ZIFT. If current research on transcervical tubal cannulation shows that GIFT and ZIFT can be done *nonsurgically* with the same success rates achieved using laparoscopy, these techniques will continue to play a role pending improvements in the IVF laboratory.

Embryo implantation

It has been somewhat surprising that more transferred embryos do not implant. One recent clue has been the finding that embryos which are more likely to implant have areas of thinning of the zona, which may help them to hatch (or break out of) this protective shell to begin to burrow into the endometrium. A second clue is that when a hole is made in the shell to assist fertilization, the chance of implantation seems to increase. One researcher is therefore making a small hole in the shell before transfer, which he calls "assisting hatching." Preliminary results show a significant boost in the number of embryos leading to clinical pregnancies. If this proves out, it appears that some embryos fail to develop because they are unable to secrete enough enzymes to thin the shell adequately. It is this sort of leap forward that could certainly lead, together with other refinements, to a doubling of the success rate.

Embryo freezing

Embryo freezing has come a long way in the last few years. Further developments combined with improved stimulation will lead to a boost of the pregnancy rate per retrieval above what we see at present. The occurrence of more than one pregnancy with a single retrieval, as seen with the Mohr "triplets" (conceived at the same time but born years apart), will become commonplace.

Sperm preparation

Advances in sperm preparation will gradually reduce the incidence of failed or reduced fertilization.

Better diagnostic tests

Advances in diagnosis will allow better recognition of cases where the male or female gametes are of such reduced quality that the outcome of the IVF cycle is destined to be poor. Use of frozen donor sperm restores the outcome to normal, whereas egg donation doubles the rate over routine IVF. Given an adequate supply of donors, the use of egg donation will greatly expand for older women, for those who stimulate poorly, and for couples with failed IVF cycles who wish to raise their chance of success to a much higher level.

Genetic engineering

In the more distant future, it is quite probable that hereditary defects will be rectified by genetic engineering techniques to allow couples with a increased risk of genetically defective offspring to have their own normal child without having to resort to donated gametes.

Genetic screening

One of the most frequent questions we are asked is if we can tell if an embryo is a boy or a girl or, in fact, is normal. So far, the answer has been no. In as little as four to six years, though, it is predicted that genetic testing and diagnosis of embryos with diseases caused by a single gene defect may be possible. The diseases which are likely candidates for screening are Tay-Sachs disease, one type of muscular dystrophy, Huntington's chorea, and cystic fibrosis. Several of these diseases can already be detected prenatally and the number keeps on rising. As of the tenth International Workshop on Human Gene Mapping, the official number of genes tracked to specific sites on human chromosomes grew to 1700. Among the recent mapped genes that cause human disease are:

- The gene that accounts for 50 percent of the genetic susceptibility to insulin-dependent diabetes
- One that may play a role in connective-tissue diseases such as rheumatoid arthritis
- A gene that may be important in treating depression

The biggest obstacle to the development of this technology is the difficulty of obtaining DNA from such an early embryo without damaging the embryo. This would probably require development of the embryo to a further (blastocyst) stage and cryopreservation until the tests could be completed. This technology will not improve success rates, but it will make IVF safer for couples with a family history of some of the more common genetic diseases. One by-product of genetic testing would be sex determination of the embryo.

Fertilization enhancement

One of the most intensive areas for research has been the attempt to improve fertilization rates by performing procedures to open the zona of the egg for the penetration of a sperm. These techniques are known as micromanipulation and zona drilling. The opening of the zona can be achieved either by dissection with microsurgical techniques or by digestion with enzymes.

It has been found that the use of enzymes may cause damage to the embryos and so the most promising method is now partial zona dissection (PZD), where a microscopic incision is made in the zona using only mechanical force with a glass needle. This enhances fertilization in couples with a severe male factor problem. First the egg is shrunk by means of a sugar solution to allow room to puncture the shell without damaging the egg. Then the egg is held steady with a micromanipulator and a tiny glass needle pierces the shell, leaving a small opening for the sperm to enter. However, in addition to promoting fertilization with a single sperm, the incision in the zona removes some of the egg's protection from fertilization with more than one sperm (polyspermy), which is reported to occur in about 20 percent of PZD cases. Polyspermic eggs are abnormal and must be discarded.

Researchers at Emory University in Atlanta recently produced five pregnancies utilizing PZD in couples with a male factor problem. PZD is claimed by the Atlanta physicians to approximately double the fertilization rate in such couples (from 30 percent to 60 percent). It is reassuring that animal studies have shown that there is no greater incidence of birth defects in offspring from dissected eggs. If this new technique reaches its potential, it could dramatically increase pregnancy rates in a group of patients for whom there is no other specific therapy, and that will have an effect on overall pregnancy rates.

Cryopreservation

Embryo freezing is an area that has the greatest potential to result in much better pregnancy rates per stimulation and retrieval. Better freezing techniques can also result in a lower rate of multiple pregnancies since physicians will not feel so pressed to transfer larger number of embryos during the IVF cycle itself, rather than freezing more of the apparently good-quality embryos for transfer in future cycles. Currently it appears that the ability of the embryo to survive is reduced by about half by the effects of freezing.

CONSUMER ISSUES

As we indicated at the outset, some serious consumer issues need attention:

- The general lack of insurance reimbursement for infertility treatment and, specifically, assisted reproductive procedures
- The lack of any professional or governmental oversight of IVF clinics and laboratories
- The lack of universal definitions of qualifications for physicians and technicians performing these procedures
- The dearth of any objective information by which the consumer can compare programs and make an informed selection, except for the March 1989 congressional survey
- Misleading advertising
- The high cost of these procedures

To their credit, Congressman Ron Wyden and the subcommittee did a credible job in bringing these issues to the forefront and providing the public its first unbiased comparison between many of the IVF and GIFT programs in the United States. But the progress should not stop here.

LACK OF INSURANCE. Infertility is a medical problem that can devastate a family no less than any other serious medical condition. Sure, you don't die from infertility. But we are now providing coverage for many other nonlethal medical conditions, and infertility coverage should be mandated by law. Some states have or are in the process of passing such laws. IVF and GIFT are now accepted clinical procedures and are no longer experimental. Insurance should provide coverage for a reasonable number of cycles in couples who have not been able to achieve pregnancy by other conventional means.

LACK OF OVERSIGHT. Several of the prominent physicians who testified before the congressional subcommittee addressed the issue of oversight. Dr. Richard Marrs, director of the Institute for Reproductive Research at the Hospital of the Good Samaritan in Los Angeles, suggested: "Laboratories providing and performing tests or evaluations of oocyte or gamete function should be licensed just like any other diagnostic laboratory, on a state-to-state basis. Laboratories that perform GIFT, IVF, ZIFT, and TE(S)T, all these new reproductive processes that are coming down the pike, embryo freezing, anything that we are doing now or in the future should also be licensed."

Dr. Alan H. deCherney, professor of obstetrics and gynecology at Yale University and a member of the board of directors of the American Fertility Society (AFS) also endorsed regulation of laboratories and felt that gamete laboratories should come under the same state-by-state scrutiny as other laboratories. He felt that the British system, where a voluntary licensing authority is made up of physicians and other members of society to "inspect and scrutinize" IVF centers, could be used as a model for this country. But as of now there still is no regulatory mechanism for IVF centers, just a promise from Rep. Wyden to introduce legislation to regulate embryo laboratories.

QUALIFICATIONS. We are also no closer to a definition of qualifications for claiming expertise in infertility or performing high-tech reproductive procedures. Actually, this situation is no different than other areas of medicine. When physicians are issued a state license, they can claim to be expert in any field and limit their practice to that field. In general, policing of qualifications has been delegated to the hospital medical staffs. But if a hospital would allow it, any physician theoretically could do neurosurgery or heart transplants, not to mention ART procedures, without any formal training. (Review Chapter 8 for clues to ensure that the doctor treating you has proper qualifications.) On the other hand, it does take knowledge and work to find that out. One valuable resource for determining qualifications is the AFS's booklet "Questions to Ask About IVF and GIFT Programs."

OBJECTIVE INFORMATION. The March 9, 1989, hearing by the subcommittee released to the public, for the first time, a survey comparing the centers that voluntarily chose to report their results.

However, there are some problems with the data. As we explain in detail in Appendix 1, some programs misinterpreted a question and consequently reported higher-than-achieved pregnancy rates for 1988, and, as subcommittee Chairman Wyden stated, the results may somewhat reflect the difficulty of cases performed by a particular center. More difficult problems such as male factor, older women, or couples failing treatment in other centers will adversely affect a program's success rate.

So what about reporting in the future? The congressional survey was a one-time study. Soon these 1987 and 1988 surveys will be history, and changes in personnel and techniques can result in dramatic changes in success in a short period of time. No mechanism exists for a continuing survey. The Society of Assisted Reproductive Technology continues to collect data but only releases an annual report on assisted reproduction in general. As you are aware by now, you cannot apply general data to a specific center. According to testimony by Dr. Stuart Hartz, president of Medical Research International, which designed and conducts the IVF registry started by the American Fertility Society and SART, it was determined at the outset that "the data submitted by each clinic would remain confidential and would be published as pooled or summary statistics." It was felt that the confidentiality helps to "minimize biased reporting" since the registry does not have enough resources to audit the information. This method of collection of data does have great scientific importance, but it would be a shame to have virtually all the programs in the country (135) now reporting without the individual data available for public use. Fortunately, the majority of SART members have recently indicated their support for continuing to supply clinic-specific data similar to the congressional survey.

ADVERTISING. Dr. deCherney testified: "Infertility patients are exceptionally vulnerable to exploitation. No one dies. As mentioned, success rates are not high; therefore failure rates are difficult to assess. More importantly, though, patients are desperate to have children and will go to any length to accomplish this goal." He felt that "some exploitation of patients by physicians in the field of infertility medicine does exist. . . . The magnitude of this is not known. . . . My estimate is that it is proportionally quite small." In reviewing much of the promotional material from centers from all over the country, we find that most of it is accurate and straightforward. As in any field, you will find those who stray from the bounds of total accuracy, but we feel that consumer awareness is the best mechanism for dealing with these improprieties.

We are not optimistic that government regulation ever will exert real authority over advertising practices in this country except for blatant examples. Rep. Wyden apparently agrees with us; he told *The New York Times*: "We are looking upon the professional societies, such as the American Fertility Society, to establish professional standards and to develop guidelines for advertising and ethics."

COSTS. The congressional hearing did not consider the issue of costs of these procedures. They are very expensive. But when you put them into the perspective of other high-tech procedures such as MRI scans, transplants, or even conventional surgery such as a hysterectomy or gall bladder operation, the costs of ART procedures are quite reasonable considering what is involved. A rough breakdown of costs for an "average cycle" today would be about:

Medications	$1700 ±
Monitoring ovulation	$1000
Retrieval procedure	$2200 ±
Laboratory costs for fertilization	$1000
Transfer	$ 300
Embryo freezing	$ 350

It may not surprise you to learn that we don't expect them to go down considerably. Nevertheless, they probably won't go up much either unless new technology makes the procedure more complicated, as in the case that needs zona drilling. We feel that the increasing numbers of programs will create a competitive market, which will tend to stabilize prices.

GOING OUT ON A LIMB

What all this boils down to is "What will the success rate be twelve years from now when the field of ART will reach almost the quarter-century mark?" Dr. Gary Hodgen feels we will double our present success rates in seven to eight years. With all the above developments, it is possible that the term-pregnancy rate per egg retrieval could approach 50 percent. In that case, surgery for all except ligated tubes may be relegated to the Dark Ages and we'll tell our young colleagues that we actually used to try to fix damaged tubes.

"Test-tube babies" will be so commonplace that the procedure won't be thought of as unusual, but rather as simply one of the many highly successful infertility treatments available to couples to fulfill their potential to have a family.

Appendix one

Congressional Survey Results

Some Words of Caution

Finally there is some way to compare IVF centers. Right? Well, maybe. With some knowledge about what the figures mean you can make a reasonably well-informed choice, but there are several deficiencies in the report you must be aware of before you accept the numbers at face value.

First, if you want to read the entire report you'll find out how to obtain it in Appendix 3. But when you read it, ignore the advertising. Yes, advertising! Why the compilers of the report allowed some programs to put in reams of promotional material without giving everyone the opportunity is beyond comprehension, particularly when the whole point of the report was to provide objective information.

Second, there was an unfortunate major error in the structure of the questionnaire on which the report was based. It asked for all the IVF deliveries, for example, in 1988. Some programs gave a figure for all IVF patients who delivered in 1988 *even if they had had their procedure in 1987*. For these programs the number of pregnancies for 1988 includes not only all of those for the 1988 cycles but also many of the 1987 cycles, thus overinflating the 1988 results by as much as 15 percent or more. This appears to be the major reason why the average 1988 birth rate in the Congressional survey was higher than the 1988 IVF Registry results. The only way to get a hint which programs might have made this error is to look at the proportion of pregnancies, "continuing" versus "live births." Since the questionnaire was due December 15 (although some arrived later) and pregnancy lasts nine months, only about *one-fourth* of the 1988 pregnancies should be delivered and listed in the "live birth" category, although chance variation and preterm births may increase the percentage somewhat. If *one-half* or more were delivered, we suggest you *confirm with that program how many cycles were done in 1988 and how many live births occurred from those cycles.* You certainly don't want to choose a less convenient program unless it is clearly more successful. A third inconsistency is that some programs may have included pregnancies that occurred from frozen embryos from those cycles, but this would account for less than a 5 percent increase.

Another deficiency is that there was no strong caution about the fact that percentages were based in many cases on a small number of cycles. Giving a rate on fewer than ten cycles is almost meaningless, but even with fifty cycles, there is enormous variability based on chance alone. For example, with fifty cycles and a "success rate" of 15 percent, the actual rate based on their techniques in a thousand cases could vary anywhere from 5 percent to 25 percent, and the 15 percent they obtained was simply based on the fertility potential (with this procedure) of the fifty men and women who happened to go through the procedures at that time. Even with 200 cases, the 95 percent confidence limits of a 15 percent success rate is 10 percent to 20 percent. This is why programs experience such wide swings of success rate from time to time; it's simply the chance variation of the inherent fertility potential of the couples treated, as expected from simple statistical calculations. So, if you want to pick a program in which you can have a reasonable estimate of the true success rate, consider only those with a combined total of at least 100 to 200 cases in the two years or at least 100 cases for a single year.

Given these caveats, there is still one more very big factor. Are the patients really comparable from one program to another? Unfortunately, the answer is only a qualified "maybe."

In the first place, a new program is wise not to take on difficult cases until those running it are sure everything is going well. You don't need to wonder if the fertilization rate is low because of some problem in the laboratory. At one of the early conferences several years ago comprised of the heads of the various IVF programs beginning around the country, one of the directors, who had good results to report but has never done remotely as well since that time, said, "Of course we chose these patients to be ideal." He then paused and looked around the room and added, "Didn't everyone?" So, if you are considering a new program that has small numbers, you are taking a double risk. A short-term rate of even 30 percent or 40 percent could actually be, over the long haul, compatible with a true rate of 5 percent to 10 percent.

At the other extreme, programs that are well known for their expertise tend to gather patients who are concerned about associated problems or their lack of success in other programs and seek out "the best" to maximize their chance of success. The following is a sampling of some difficult patients coming into our program as an illustration of this phenomenon:

- L. L.—seven failed IVF cycles
- A. S.—age forty, four failed IVF attempts
- J. M.—five failed IVF cycles
- T. K.—two failed IVF cycles with zero to low fertilization rate
- R. T.—age forty, four failed IVF and one failed GIFT cycle with zero to low fertilization rate.
- G. W.—four failed IVF cycles with zero to low fertilization rate
- E. W.—four failed IVF cycles
- F. M.—three failed cycles with low fertilization rate
- R. C.—four failed IVF cycles

How can you adjust for this variable? You wouldn't be far off if you subtracted 10 percent for new programs and added 5 percent for well-recognized programs as a rule of thumb.

How about age? Some programs accept women older than those admitted by others. This has a relatively small but significant impact. If you are under forty-one, look at the actual questionnaire in the full congressional report for the percent of women over forty-one in the particular program you are interested in. For each 5 percent of women over forty-one, add 1 percent to the term pregnancy rate (for most programs this will be about 1 percent to 2 percent). This will allow you to cancel out this difference among programs, but you will find that, with rare exceptions, it will only account for a 1 percent to 2 percent variation among different programs.

The final major variable in patient selection depends upon whether it is assured that all other reasonable fertility therapy, including adequate time, has been applied. If so, many of the most fertile women have been removed from the IVF population. For example, for several years we have recommended Pergonal combined with intrauterine insemination for women with open and reasonably normal tubes before going on to an ART procedure. This has resulted in numerous pregnancies, and we have no doubt that these women would have had a very good chance of being counted among the successes if they had gone directly to IVF or GIFT. For a patient choosing a program, this is a difficult variable to assess. You are probably better off in a program that does IVF as part of a general infertility service. Also, becoming a well-informed consumer by reading a book such as this one will help you assure that *everything else* has been tried before resorting to ART procedures. If an ART procedure is being suggested, ask why any treatment that seems to apply to you has not been done. Ask what your chance of pregnancy will be if you simply take more time. If ART is being suggested prematurely, you may want to adjust down that program's success rate by 10 percent. Remember, one underlying principle is to always try to achieve pregnancy in the simplist, least expensive way with the least risk. That should be your goal, too, although being impatient because of age, duration of infertility, or other personal factors is understandable. You may choose to bypass one of the options offered to you, but it is important that it should be a well-informed choice.

It is also good to remember that convenience, personal attention, and program organization will influence your chance of success. If the process is not easily tolerated and you decide to quit after one cycle instead of three or four, your chance of success will have been greatly affected. At the same time beware of programs that make it too simple; there is just no simple way to a high rate of success. The best way to evaluate this factor is to have a recommendation from a satisfied patient or from a physician whose patients have been happy with the care they received.

If you are already in a program that satisfies the above criteria we *do not* advise switching merely because *you* have not been successful. It is expected in the best program that most patients will require multiple attempts. The loss of continuity may deprive you of the "experience factor" whereby physicians and laboratory personnel can make subtle adjustments to improve your chance of success. Also, you will lose the "comfort factor" in being familiar with the team members who have been caring for you already.

This all may sound complicated, but it's worth the effort. By the way, the couple with the seven previous attempts conceived on their first cycle. You can be sure they wished they had been able to make a better initial choice based on all the information here.

INTERPRETING THE SURVEY RESULTS

We categorized the results of the congressional survey into seven categories for each center in two tables, one for IVF and another for GIFT. The 1987 and 1988 results are presented for each category. The categories are:

1. YEARS: Number of years the center has been in operation for these procedures prior to December 31, 1988.
2. STIM CYCLES: Number of stimulation cycles in an attempt to produce multiple eggs in the woman.
3. EGG RET: Number of cycles in which an attempt was made to retrieve eggs.
4. LIVE: Number of live births. All of the successful pregnancies should be reported in this category for 1987. Less than half the pregnancies for 1988 should be in this category or we would suspect the program misinterpreted the questionnaire and may have included pregnancies conceived in 1987 which delivered in 1988, inflating their success rate. If close to or more than half the pregnancies for 1988 fall into this category, discuss this with the program before accepting success rates based on these data at face value.
5. CONT PREG: Pregnancies that are ongoing but have not yet resulted in a birth. This number should be 0 for 1987, since all patients conceived in 1987 should have delivered by the date this questionnaire was due. The majority of pregnancies for 1988 should fall into this category.

In the 1988 data, some pregnancies conceived toward the end of the year will be very early. Some of these may not result in term pregnancy. In a program with a substantial volume this will have a limited effect on the term pregnancy rate, since most pregnancies conceived in 1988 would be beyond twelve weeks. In programs with limited volume, miscarriage of that early pregnancy could substantially alter the term pregnancy rate, if the pregnancies clustered toward the end of 1988, by chance or because the program was new or improving.

6. L + C/ER: Success rate based on the number of egg retrievals that resulted in a live birth or continuing pregnancy. Data reported as — in this column indicate that no cases were done in the year being reported; see comments under 5.

7. L + C/SC: Success rate based on the number of stimulated cycles that resulted in a live birth or continuing pregnancy. Data reported as — in this column indicate that no cases were done in the year being reported; see comments under 5.

WARNING: DO NOT REFER TO THE TABLES WITHOUT READING THE INTRODUCTION ("Some Words of Caution") TO THIS APPENDIX. Several factors make comparisons among the raw numbers quite hazardous. The tables in the congressional report contained some inconsistencies which we attempted to correct by using data directly from the questionnaires. We cannot be responsible for the accuracy of these data and recommend that you obtain a copy of the subcommittee report for complete information. Where there may be a question, contact each center you are considering directly to clarify any inconsistencies and learn of their recent experience. Refer to Appendix 2 for the full names and addresses of each program and the address from which to obtain a copy of the subcommittee report.

Adapted from the hearing before the Subcommittee on Regulation, Business opportunities, and Energy of the Committee on Small Business—House of Representatives, Washington, D.C., March 9, 1989

IVF DATA

PROGRAM	YEARS	87/88 STIM CYCLES	87/88 EGG RET	87/88 LIVE	87/88 CONT PREG	87/88 L+C/ER	87/88 L+C/SC
	(1)	(2)	(3)	(4)	(5)	(6)	(7)
ALABAMA							
Assisted Reproductive	2.2	268/219	227/181	34/19	00/08	15/15	13/12
Univ. of Al.-Birmingham	5.0	53/ 39	30/ 21	01/00	00/04	03/19	02/10
Univ. of South Alabama	1.6	17/ 22	17/ 21	00/00	00/00	00/00	00/00
ARIZONA							
Az. Cent. Fert. Studies	4.6	NA/NA	07/ 05	00/00	00/00	00/00	NA/NA
Az. Fertility Institute	5.0	81/117	72/108	12/04	00/08	17/11	15/10
Az. Repro. Inst. of Tucson	3.0	08/ 10	07/ 09	00/00	00/01	00/11	00/10
Southwest Fertility	0.5	00/ 06	00/ 04	00/00	00/01	—/25	—/17
CALIFORNIA							
Alta Bates Hospital	5.0	137/141	109/114	17/13	00/14	16/24	12/19
AMI-South Bay Hospital	2.0	115/147	99/122	25/09	00/20	25/24	22/20
Cal.-Irvine IVF-GIFT	2.5	239/263	163/188	27/04	00/25	17/15	11/11
Cedars-Sinai Med Center	2.4	00/136	00/ 90	00/06	00/08	—/16	—/10
Central Ca. IVF Program	4.0	60/106	54/ 86	06/03	00/10	11/15	10/14
Century City Hosp.	6.0	89/185	89/152	02/11	00/18	02/19	02/16

IVF DATA

PROGRAM	YEARS	87/88 STIM CYCLES	87/88 EGG RET	87/88 LIVE	87/88 CONT PREG	87/88 L+C/ER	87/88 L+C/SC
	(1)	(2)	(3)	(4)	(5)	(6)	(7)
Fert & Repro Health	0.2	00/ 13	00/ 13	00/00	00/05	—/38	—/38
Forest Fertility Center	1.0	00/ 09	00/ 09	00/00	00/01	00/11	—/11
Hoag Fertility Service	1.2	12/ 52	04/ 29	00/03	00/06	00/31	00/17
Hosp. of Good Sam.	8.0	402/208	304/149	31/00	00/19	10/13	08/09
Huntington Repro. Ctr.	0.5	00/ 68	00/ 53	00/00	00/08	—/15	—/12
Infertil Med Group-San Diego	6.0	147/113	101/ 87	06/01	00/04	06/06	04/04
John Muir Memorial	4.7	718/390	365/300	64/16	00/47	18/21	09/16
North. Calif. Fert.	6.0	76/ 42	46/ 30	05/00	00/04	11/13	07/10
Northridge Hosp.	4.5	257/185	180/152	24/26	00/12	13/25	09/21
Nova Fertility Center	1.2	05/ 80	05/ 54	00/04	01/09	20/30	20/20
Pacific Fertility Cen.	1.0	00/123	00/102	00/06	00/16	—/22	—/18
S. Cal. Fertility Ins.	4.0	20/ 17	17/ 12	00/01	00/02	00/25	00/18
Stanford University	3.0	121/ 64	83/ 49	00/00	00/02	00/04	00/03
UCLA Medical Center	5.3	152/105	122/ 98	22/08	00/08	18/16	14/15
UCSF Fertility Assoc.	6.0	194/215	124/142	11/06	00/20	09/18	06/12
USC School of Med.	2.5	113/161	84/146	10/10	00/15	12/17	09/16
Whittier Hospital	1.0	00/ 13	00/ 08	00/00	00/01	—/13	—/08
COLORADO							
Inf/Gyn/Obs-Englewood	0.8	00/ 54	00/ 50	00/00	00/14	—/28	—/25
Reproductive Genetics	6.3	173/254	130/200	13/10	00/14	10/12	08/09

CONNECTICUT							
Mt. Sinai Hospital	4.6	45/ 47	26/ 39	02/01	00/02	08/08	04/06
UCONN School of Med.	6.0	67/ 89	34/ 47	02/03	00/03	06/13	03/07
Yale School of Med.	6.6	473/466	381/342	32/23	00/14	08/11	07/08
DELEWARE							
Repro. Endo and Fert.-Newark	0.8	00/118	00/ 70	00/00	00/04	—/06	—/03
D.C. (WASHINGTON)							
Columbia Hos. for Wom.	2.0	00/162	00/134	00/04	00/15	—/14	—/12
GW University IVF	6.0	12/ 61	11/ 50	01/01	00/09	09/20	08/16
FLORIDA							
Fert. Cen. of Boca Raton	1.1	04/ 35	02/ 31	00/01	00/03	00/13	00/11
Florida Fertility	1.4	18/ 20	16/ 12	00/00	00/00	00/00	00/00
Humana Women's Hosp.	3.0	62/ 89	44/ 59	06/06	00/06	14/20	10/13
Jacksonville Mem. Med.	2.6	19/ 14	15/ 09	01/01	00/01	07/22	05/14
N.W. Fla. Gulf Breeze	1.3	14/ 36	12/ 31	00/02	00/04	00/19	00/17
NW Center for Infert.	1.4	28/106	20/ 70	00/03	03/06	15/13	11/08
Park Ave. Women's Centr.	0.2	00/ 07	00/ 00	00/07	00/01	—/—	—/14
Sand Lake IVF Center.	2.5	89/143	74/114	10/09	00/11	14/18	11/14
University of Miami	6.0	75/ 52	68/ 43	03/02	00/03	04/12	04/10
GEORGIA							
Augusta Reprod. Bio.	5.0	25/ 36	24/ 32	01/05	04/07	21/38	20/33
Med. College of Ga.	4.0	25/ 35	14/ 19	03/00	00/01	21/05	12/03
Reproductive Biology	6.0	224/329	156/227	29/11	00/45	19/25	13/17

IVF DATA

PROGRAM	YEARS (1)	87/88 STIM CYCLES (2)	87/88 EGG RET (3)	87/88 LIVE (4)	87/88 CONT PREG (5)	87/88 L+C/ER (6)	87/88 L+C/SC (7)
HAWAII							
Kauai Med. Group	4.0	00/ 05	00/ 05	00/00	00/00	—/00	—/00
Pacific IVF Institute	3.6	37/120	27/ 88	05/10	00/08	19/20	14/15
ILLINOIS							
Evanston and Glenbrook	2.0	00/110	00/100	00/05	00/15	—/20	—/18
Masonic Medical Cent.	2.1	86/117	61/ 90	02/04	00/09	03/14	02/11
Michael Reese Hospital	6.0	108/128	109/132	04/01	00/05	04/05	04/05
Northwestern Memorial	2.0	35/ 18	27/ 11	00/04	00/01	00/45	00/28
Rush Presb-St. Luke's	5.1	77/ 72	77/ 72	07/02	00/05	09/10	09/10
Mt. Sinai-Chicago	6.0	53/ 72	34/ 66	01/03	00/09	03/18	02/16
Un. of Illinois Med. Cen.	4.2	14/ 07	09/ 05	00/00	00/00	00/00	00/00
INDIANA							
Center for Reprod.	1.4	22/ 37	12/ 35	00/00	00/03	00/09	00/08
Indiana University	6.0	01/ 03	00/ 02	00/00	00/00	—/00	00/00
Pregnancy Initiation	3.0	201/210	152/151	12/08	00/11	08/13	06/09
IOWA							
University of Iowa	1.8	22/ 88	17/ 62	00/00	00/10	00/16	00/11

Facility							
KANSAS							
Reprod. Resource Cen.	1.3	89/121	68/ 97	01/12	00/11	01/24	01/19
Univ. Kansas Wichita	1.6	24/ 22	16/ 14	00/01	00/05	00/43	00/27
KENTUCKY							
Fertility Institute	2.1	10/ 01	10/ 01	00/00	00/00	00/00	00/00
Norton Hospital	5.0	57/ 66	49/ 62	04/08	08/09	24/27	21/26
University of Kentucky	3.5	46/ 79	26/ 59	02/02	00/04	08/10	04/08
LOUISIANA							
Fertility Center-Kenner	1.5	119/105	101/ 91	15/12	00/08	15/19	30/26
Fertility Inst. New Orleans	6.0	166/ 78	98/ 67	20/04	00/10	20/21	12/18
MARYLAND							
Beth Israel-Boston	0.7	00/103	00/ 94	00/01	00/08	—/10	—/09
Ctr. for Reprod. Studies-Balt.	6.0	94/ 80	75/ 62	01/05	00/02	01/11	01/09
Johns Hopkins	4.5	81/ 96	59/ 76	NA/NA	NA/NA	NA/NA	NA/NA
Montgomery Inf. Inst.	5.0	46/ 68	47/ 68	05/02	00/03	11/07	11/07
University of Maryland	0.3	00/ 03	00/ 02	00/00	00/00	—/00	—/00
Women's Hosp. Center	4.3	440/354	440/354	61/24	00/48	14/20	14/20
MASSACHUSETTS							
Atlanticare Fertility	5.0	223/291	147/183	08/09	00/10	05/11	04/07
Boston IVF	1.2	93/333	61/294	03/04	00/16	05/07	03/06
Brigham & Women's Hosp.	6.0	94/131	65/ 73	02/14	00/08	03/30	02/17
New England Med. Centr.	0.8	00/.17	00/ 16	00/00	00/02	—/13	—/12

IVF DATA

PROGRAM	YEARS	87/88 STIM CYCLES	87/88 EGG RET	87/88 LIVE	87/88 CONT PREG	87/88 L+C/ER	87/88 L+C/SC
	(1)	(2)	(3)	(4)	(5)	(6)	(7)
MICHIGAN							
Blodgett Memorial IVF	5.4	43/ 51	39/ 44	08/08	00/05	21/30	19/25
Hutzel Hosp./Wayne St.	5.5	162/112	124/ 92	11/02	00/04	09/07	07/05
Oakwood Hospital	0.1	00/ 01	00/ 01	00/00	00/00	—/00	—/00
Schi Reprod. Endo.	1.6	49/ 79	41/ 74	04/02	00/10	10/16	08/15
Univ. Mi. Med. Centr.	5.0	75/ 83	60/ 61	03/02	00/03	05/08	04/06
William Beaumont Hosp.	5.5	115/153	100/119	10/02	00/07	10/08	09/06
MINNESOTA							
U. of Minnesota	6.0	72/139	52/103	09/02	00/10	17/12	13/09
MISSISSIPPI							
U. Miss Med. Center	5.0	85/ 65	53/ 48	12/02	00/06	23/17	14/12
MISSOURI							
Washington U. Jewish	6.0	77/ 97	53/ 55	05/04	00/02	09/11	06/06
NEBRASKA							
Methodist Hospital	1.6	10/ 19	11/ 17	00/00	00/02	00/12	00/11
University of Nebraska	1.0	00/ 50	00/ 40	00/01	00/01	—/05	—/05
NEVADA							
Northern Nv. Fertility	6.0	188/155	139/123	17/08	00/14	12/18	09/14

NEW HAMPSHIRE							
Dartmouth-Hitchcock	08/20	11/33	00/01	01/01	09/ 06	12/ 10	3.0
NEW JERSEY							
Robert Wood Johnson	07/07	12/13	00/02	09/11	76/101	128/182	5.5
UMDNJ NJ Med Schools	07/09	09/10	00/09	12/06	139/156	162/166	2.7
NEW MEXICO							
Presbyterian IVF	—/15	—/17	00/04	00/01	00/ 29	00/ 34	2.0
NEW YORK							
Albert Einstein Coll.	06/09	09/11	02/06	02/00	47/ 55	67/ 67	2.6
Australia United Hosp.	13/15	16/17	00/120	107/20	650/807	805/957	2.7
Children's Hos. (Buff.)	—/00	—/00	00/00	00/00	00/ 22	00/ 30	1.0
Columbia Presbyterian	00/17	00/22	00/04	00/08	55/ 54	69/ 71	5.8
Life Program	—/00	—/00	00/00	00/00	00/ 15	00/ 15	0.6
Long Island IVF	—/21	—/24	00/27	00/00	00/114	00/127	1.0
Mt. Sinai Hospital	08/17	11/19	00/31	21/33	193/330	267/369	2.1
NY Hospital-Cornell	07/08	11/11	00/24	13/02	116/244	175/313	2.0
SUNY-Syracuse	—/00	—/00	00/00	00/00	00/ 08	00/NA	0.6
St. Luke's Roosevelt	11/00	18/00	02/00	02/00	22/ 20	36/ 33	4.0
U. of Rochester CARE	04/08	05/08	00/04	03/01	61/ 60	72/ 63	5.5
Wayne Decker IVF Program	00/09	00/14	00/04	00/01	11/ 37	15/ 53	1.6
NORTH CAROLINA							
Duke University Med.	06/08	08/12	00/05	04/01	50/ 52	71/ 75	6.0
NC Memorial Hospital	14/—	21/—	12/00	15/00	127/ 00	195/ 00	6.0
N.C. Reprod. Center	17/25	17/40	00/02	01/00	06/ 05	06/ 08	1.7

IVF DATA

PROGRAM	YEARS	87/88 STIM CYCLES	87/88 EGG RET	87/88 LIVE	87/88 CONT PREG	87/88 L+C/ER	87/88 L+C/SC
	(1)	(2)	(3)	(4)	(5)	(6)	(7)
OHIO							
Akron City Hospital	3.5	70/ 90	44/ 52	02/10	01/10	07/38	04/22
Bethesda Fertility	1.5	07/ 48	05/ 41	01/00	00/05	20/12	14/10
Cleveland Clinic Found.	4.1	176/141	149/112	11/10	00/06	07/14	06/11
Fertility Inst.-Cincinnati	2.1	10/ 01	10/ 01	00/00	00/00	00/00	00/00
Jewish Hosp. of Cin.	5.1	07/ 05	03/ 05	00/00	00/01	00/20	00/20
MacDonald Hospital	4.1	44/ 96	22/ 50	02/00	00/05	09/10	05/05
Miami Valley Hospital	4.6	100/ 45	69/ 41	05/02	00/03	07/12	05/11
Midwest Reprod. Inst.	5.0	37/ 43	26/ 27	00/00	00/02	00/07	00/05
Mt. Sinai Med. Center	6.0	71/ 59	49/ 48	04/02	00/04	08/13	06/10
Ohio State	6.3	105/136	79/102	06/04	00/02	08/06	06/04
Riverside Reprod. Serv.	1.2	12/ 51	10/ 38	00/01	00/01	00/05	00/04
Univ. Reprod. Center	6.3	105/136	79/102	06/04	00/02	08/06	06/04
OKLAHOMA							
Henry Bennett Fertility	2.7	24/ 31	23/ 19	03/01	00/00	08/05	06/03
Hillcrest Fertility	6.0	46/ 52	40/ 50	02/00	00/07	05/14	04/13
OREGON							
Emanuel Hospital	1.6	29/ 66	27/ 54	04/02	00/04	15/11	14/09
Or. Health Science U.	5.6	77/ 63	49/ 53	03/03	00/09	06/23	04/19

PENNSYLVANIA							
Albert Einstein Med.	3.9	45/ 67	38/ 57	06/03	00/03	16/11	13/09
Christian Fert Inst.-Easton	3.0	90/107	90/106	05/14	08/08	14/21	14/21
Endocrine Hist. Assoc.	1.0	00/211	00/200	00/01	00/16	—/08	—/08
Fert. Ctr. St. Lukes	2.0	00/ 10	06/ 10	00/00	00/00	00/—	—/00
Hospital of U. Penn.	6.5	228/310	186/264	19/14	00/24	10/14	08/12
Magee-Women's Hospital	6.0	50/139	32/100	00/03	00/12	00/15	00/11
Penn. Repro. Assoc.	5.3	354/479	281/369	31/12	00/33	11/12	09/09
Pittsburgh Institute	1.2	05/ 12	05/ 10	00/00	00/02	00/20	00/17
Women's Clinic Ltd.	2.1	45/ 69	36/ 60	05/03	00/04	14/12	11/10
RHODE ISLAND							
Women's & Infants Hosp.	1.8	09/ 14	09/ 13	00/00	00/03	00/23	00/21
SOUTH CAROLINA							
MUSC IVF Program	4.2	15/ 13	11/ 11	00/02	01/01	09/27	07/23
Southeastern Fertility	5.0	50/ 82	27/ 41	01/01	00/01	04/05	02/02
TENNESSEE							
E. Tenn. State. Univ.	2.7	24/ 14	21/ 12	00/00	00/01	00/08	00/07
Pair (Memphis)	0.2	00/ 14	00/ 12	00/00	00/00	—/00	—/00
Univ. of Tenn. Knoxville	1.1	03/ 01	01/ 13	00/00	00/00	00/00	00/00
Vanderbilt Med. Centr.	7.0	127/126	99/116	11/12	00/12	11/21	09/19
TEXAS							
Baylor GIFT/IVF	5.5	249/261	159/174	07/03	00/12	04/09	03/06
Center for Repro. Med.	2.5	40/ 63	34/ 56	00/05	00/03	00/14	00/13
Ft. Worth Infert. Ctr.	3.7	66/ 85	31/ 37	02/01	00/01	06/05	03/02

IVF DATA

PROGRAM	YEARS	87/88 STIM CYCLES	87/88 EGG RET	87/88 LIVE	87/88 CONT PREG	87/88 L+C/ER	87/88 L+C/SC
	(1)	(2)	(3)	(4)	(5)	(6)	(7)
Houston Reproductive	5.0	02/ 21	06/ 16	00/00	00/04	00/25	00/19
J. B. Belue, M.D.	0.0	00/ 00	00/ 00	00/00	00/00	—/—	—/—
OB & GYN Associates	6.0	103/190	82/170	14/13	00/26	17/23	14/21
Presb. Hosp. Dallas	4.6	09/ 03	03/ 02	00/00	00/00	00/00	00/00
Scott & White Clinic	0.4	00/ 04	00/ 03	00/00	00/01	—/33	00/25
St. David's-Austin	4.8	30/ 75	90/116	04/02	00/08	04/07	13/13
Trinity IVF-ET Program	6.0	56/123	66/107	10/07	00/07	15/13	18/11
U of Tx-SW Med School	4.2	14/ 30	11/ 26	00/00	00/05	00/19	00/17
U of Tx-Galveston	5.0	15/ 00	15/ 00	03/00	00/00	20/—	20/—
UTAH							
University of Utah	5.7	96/104	79/ 86	12/09	00/15	15/28	13/23
VERMONT							
University of Vermont	2.6	12/ 07	07/ 05	00/00	00/00	00/00	00/00
VIRGINIA							
Henrico Drs. Hosp.	4.6	21/ 38	14/ 30	05/04	00/04	36/27	24/21
Jones Institute	8.0	737/783	637/705	106/21	00/88	17/15	14/14
Medical College of Va.	2.1	43/ 33	26/ 30	01/10	00/06	04/53	02/48
University of Va.	2.2	08/ 03	08/ 03	00/00	00/01	00/33	00/33

WASHINGTON							
Fert Clin Puget Sound	4.0	45/ 17	39/ 17	04/00	00/01	10/06	09/06
Rice & Associates	0.8	00/ 01	00/ 03	00/00	00/00	—/00	—/00
Seattle Fert & GYN	5.0	81/120	64/ 98	08/07	00/12	13/19	10/16
Seattle Women's Clinic	1.6	04/ 01	03/ 01	00/00	00/00	00/00	00/00
Swedish Hosp. Med. Cen.	5.0	102/145	80/112	07/09	00/12	09/19	07/14
Univ. of Washington	5.0	175/195	134/139	16/10	00/12	12/16	09/11
WEST VIRGINIA							
W. Virginia Univ.	1.0	00/ 28	00/19	00/00	00/01	—/05	—/04
WISCONSIN							
Advanced Institute of Fert.	5.7	NA/NA	351/351	36/46	00/52	11/30	NA/NA
Appleton Family Fert.	2.6	11/ 08	11/ 08	01/00	00/00	09/00	09/00
Univ. of Wisconsin	6.0	69/ 78	31/ 36	02/02	00/01	06/08	03/04

Adapted from the hearing before the Subcommittee on Regulation, Business opportunities, and Energy of the Committee on Small Business-House of Representatives, Washington, D. C., March 9, 1989

GIFT DATA

PROGRAM	YEARS	87/88 STIM CYCLES	87/88 EGG RET	87/88 LIVE	87/88 CONT PREG	87/88 L+C/ER	87/88 L+C/SC
	(1)	(2)	(3)	(4)	(5)	(6)	(7)
ALABAMA							
Assisted Reproductive	0.5	00/ 08	00/ 08	00/00	00/01	—/13	—/13
Univ. of Al.-Birmingham	2.0	08/ 35	04/ 22	01/00	00/04	25/18	13/11
Univ. of South Alabama	1.2	01/ 01	01/ 01	00/00	00/00	00/00	00/00
ARIZONA							
Az. Cent. Fert. Studies	3.9	864/357	188/138	45/19	00/22	24/30	05/11
Az. Fertility Institute	4.0	12/ 01	08/ 01	01/00	00/00	13/00	08/00
Az. Repro. Inst. of Tucson	3.0	10/ 06	10/ 05	02/00	00/01	29/20	20/17
Southwest Fertility	2.1	31/ 41	16/ 21	03/01	00/03	19/19	10/10
CALIFORNIA							
Alta Bates Hospital	3.0	02/ 02	02/ 02	00/00	00/00	00/00	00/00
AMI-South Bay Hospital	1.7	03/ 03	03/ 03	01/01	00/00	33/33	33/33
Cal.-Irvine IVF-GIFT	2.5	189/248	151/156	29/10	00/30	19/26	15/16
Cedars-Sinai Med Center	2.4	00/123	00/ 82	00/19	00/02	—/26	—/17
Central Ca. IVF Program	3.0	18/ 40	09/ 28	02/02	00/08	22/36	11/25
Century City Hosp.	2.0	47/145	47/145	00/16	00/17	00/23	00/23

Fert & Repro Health	0.2	00/ 01	00/ 01	00/00	00/00	—/00	—/00
Forest Fertility Center	3.0	08/ 01	08/ 01	00/00	00/00	00/00	00/00
Hoag Fertility Service	1.2	09/ 21	04/ 07	00/00	00/03	00/43	00/14
Hosp. of Good Sam.	3.0	417/200	219/129	42/00	00/26	19/20	10/13
Huntington Repro. Ctr.	0.5	00/ 28	00/ 23	00/00	00/07	—/30	—/25
Infertil Med Group-San Diego	2.0	01/ 04	01/ 04	00/00	00/00	00/00	00/00
John Muir Memorial	3.5	22/ 14	15/ 10	03/01	00/01	20/20	14/14
North. Calif. Fert.	1.0	00/ 26	00/ 18	00/01	00/02	—/17	—/12
Northridge Hosp.	2.6	14/ 38	11/ 30	00/01	00/08	00/30	00/24
Nova Fertility Center	1.2	04/ 19	03/ 09	00/02	00/01	00/33	00/16
Pacific Fertility Cen.	0.0	00/ 00	00/ 00	00/00	00/00	—/—	—/—
S. Cal. Fertility Ins.	2.0	10/ 33	10/ 30	00/03	03/03	30/20	30/18
Stanford University	3.5	10/ 14	06/ 10	01/00	00/01	17/10	10/05
UCLA Medical Center	5.0	02/ 00	02/ 00	00/00	00/00	00/—	00/—
UCSF Fertility Assoc.	2.0	06/ 04	06/ 04	01/00	00/02	17/50	17/50
USC School of Med.	2.5	22/ 03	22/ 02	03/00	00/00	14/00	14/00
Whittier Hospital	1.0	00/ 05	00/ 04	00/00	00/02	—/50	—/40
COLORADO							
Inf/Gyn/Obs-Englewood	1.5	20/ 58	18/ 52	06/12	00/13	33/48	30/43
Reproductive Genetics	0.0	00/ 00	00/ 00	00/00	00/00	—/—	—/—
CONNECTICUT							
Mt. Sinai Hospital	1.7	05/ 07	04/ 05	00/00	00/00	00/00	00/00
UCONN School of Med.	4.0	08/ 07	08/ 07	01/00	00/00	13/00	13/00
Yale School of Med.	3.5	40/ 22	26/ 13	01/01	00/01	04/15	02/09

GIFT DATA

PROGRAM	YEARS (1)	87/88 STIM CYCLES (2)	87/88 EGG RET (3)	87/88 LIVE (4)	87/88 CONT PREG (5)	87/88 L+C/ER (6)	87/88 L+C/SC (7)
DELAWARE							
Repro. Endo and Fert.-Newark	0.8	00/ 10	00/ 06	00/00	00/02	—/33	—/20
D. C. (WASHINGTON)							
Columbia Hos. for Wom.	2.0	00/ 06	00/ 06	00/00	00/00	—/00	—/00
GW University IVF	3.0	10/ 14	10/ 14	02/00	00/05	20/36	20/36
FLORIDA							
Fert. Cen. of Boca Raton	0.8	00/ 10	00/ 09	00/00	00/00	—/00	—/00
Florida Fertility	1.5	33/ 33	28/ 29	00/07	00/05	00/41	00/36
Humana Women's Hosp.	2.2	03/ 26	02/ 19	00/01	00/06	00/37	00/27
Jacksonville Mem. Med.	1.6	33/ 20	22/ 10	01/05	00/01	05/60	03/30
N. W. Fla. Gulf Breeze	1.3	15/ 37	10/ 27	00/03	00/05	00/30	00/22
NW Center for Infert.	1.4	13/ 16	11/ 15	00/02	02/00	18/13	15/13
Park Ave. Women's Centr.	0.3	00/ 01	00/ 01	00/00	00/00	—/00	—/00
Sand Lake IVF Center.	2.1	02/ 06	02/ 06	00/00	00/01	00/17	00/17
University of Miami	4.0	08/ 12	04/ 09	00/02	00/01	00/00	33/25
GEORGIA							
Augusta Reprod. Bio.	0.0	00/ 00	00/ 00	00/00	00/00	—/—	—/—
Med. College of Ga.	2.5	01/ 04	01/ 02	00/00	00/00	00/00	00/00
Reproductive Biology	3.0	09/ 38	09/ 34	02/03	00/03	22/18	22/16

HAWAII							
Kauai Med. Group	2.0	00/ 05	00/ 05	00/00	00/00	—/00	—/00
Pacific IVF Institute	0.0	00/ 00	00/ 00	00/00	00/00	—/—	—/—
ILLINOIS							
Evanston and Glenbrook	0.6	00/ 00	00/ 10	00/00	00/03	—/30	—/30
Masonic Medical Cent.	1.0	21/ 52	15/ 34	00/06	00/05	00/32	00/21
Michael Reese Hospital	2.0	06/ 56	05/ 56	01/04	00/04	20/14	17/14
Northwestern Memorial	2.0	28/ 49	20/ 40	00/13	00/08	00/52	00/43
Rush Presb-St. Luke's	1.4	19/ 76	19/ 76	00/07	00/06	00/17	00/17
Mt. Sinai-Chicago	3.0	05/ 02	05/ 02	00/00	00/00	00/00	00/00
Un. of Illinois Med. Cen.	2.2	03/ 02	01/ 02	00/00	00/00	00/00	00/00
INDIANA							
Center for Reprod.	1.2	06/ 02	06/ 01	00/00	00/00	00/00	00/00
Indiana University	2.0	01/ 37	01/ 25	00/01	00/00	00/04	00/03
Pregnancy Initiation	3.0	282/356	192/272	20/53	00/58	10/41	07/31
IOWA							
University of Iowa	1.4	05/ 44	04/ 35	00/02	00/10	00/34	00/27
KANSAS							
Reprod. Resource Cen.	2.9	69/ 94	49/ 70	03/10	00/18	06/40	04/30
Univ. Kansas Wichita	2.0	34/ 25	27/ 20	04/02	00/02	15/20	12/16
KENTUCKY							
Fertility Institute	2.3	46/ 38	46/ 38	06/05	00/02	13/18	13/18
Norton Hospital	3.0	01/ 01	01/ 01	01/00	00/00	100/00	100/00
University of Kentucky	2.7	56/ 19	36/ 14	05/02	00/01	14/21	09/16

GIFT DATA

PROGRAM	YEARS	87/88 STIM CYCLES	87/88 EGG RET	87/88 LIVE	87/88 CONT PREG	87/88 L+C/ER	87/88 L+C/SC
	(1)	(2)	(3)	(4)	(5)	(6)	(7)
LOUISIANA							
Fertility Center-Kenner	1.5	20/ 15	20/ 15	03/02	00/00	15/13	15/13
Fertility Inst. New Orleans	4.0	288/229	144/163	26/36	00/30	18/40	09/29
MARYLAND							
Beth Israel-Boston	0.0	00/ 00	00/ 00	00/00	00/00	—/—	—/—
Ctr. for Reprod. Studies-Balt.	2.0	03/ 01	03/ 01	01/00	00/00	33/00	33/00
Johns Hopkins	3.0	04/ 08	04/ 08	NA/NA	NA/NA	NA/NA	NA/NA
Montgomery Inf. Inst.	2.5	14/ 48	14/ 48	02/04	00/05	14/19	14/19
University of Maryland	0.3	00/ 01	00/ 01	00/00	00/00	—/00	—/00
Women's Hosp. Center	2.6	23/ 36	23/ 36	03/01	00/06	13/19	13/19
MASSACHUSETTS							
Atlanticare Fertility	5.0	17/ 10	10/ 04	01/00	00/00	10/00	06/00
Boston IVF	1.2	222/342	147/260	27/15	00/33	18/18	12/14
Brigham & Women's Hosp.	3.0	09/ 09	08/ 08	01/00	00/01	13/13	11/11
New England Med. Centr.	0.5	00/ 01	00/ 01	00/00	00/00	—/00	—/00
MICHIGAN							
Blodgett Memorial IVF	0.8	00/ 05	00/ 05	00/00	00/01	—/20	—/20
Hutzel Hosp./Wayne St.	3.2	01/ 01	01/ 01	00/00	00/00	00/00	00/00
Oakwood Hospital	0.0	00/ 00	00/ 01	00/00	00/00	—/00	—/—
Schi Reprod. Endo.	1.6	45/131	42/109	10/12	00/33	24/41	22/34

Univ. Mi. Med. Centr.	3.0	02/ 04	02/ 04	00/00	00/00	00/00	00/00
William Beaumont Hosp.	2.1	02/ 06	02/ 06	01/00	00/01	50/17	50/17
MINNESOTA							
U. of Minnesota	4.0	00/ 01	00/ 01	00/00	00/01	—/100	—/100
MISSISSIPPI							
U. Miss Med. Center	4.0	02/ 04	01/ 02	01/00	00/00	100/00	50/00
MISSOURI							
Washington U. Jewish	2.0	02/ 02	02/ 02	00/00	00/00	00/00	00/00
NEBRASKA							
Methodist Hospital	1.4	04/ 01	02/ 01	00/00	00/00	00/00	00/00
University of Nebraska	0.5	00/ 04	00/ 04	00/01	00/01	—/50	—/50
NEVADA							
Northern Nv. Fertility	3.0	05/ 03	05/ 03	00/00	00/00	00/00	00/00
NEW HAMPSHIRE							
Dartmouth-Hitchcock	0.0	00/ 00	00/ 00	00/00	00/00	—/—	—/—
NEW JERSEY							
Robert Wood Johnson	3.5	00/ 13	00/ 13	00/00	00/00	—/00	—/00
UMDNJ NJ Med Schools	1.6	01/ 01	01/ 01	00/00	00/01	00/100	00/100
NEW MEXICO							
Presbyterian IVF	2.0	00/ 17	00/ 16	00/04	00/03	—/44	—/41

GIFT DATA

PROGRAM	YEARS	87/88 STIM CYCLES	87/88 EGG RET	87/88 LIVE	87/88 CONT PREG	87/88 L+C/ER	87/88 L+C/SC
	(1)	(2)	(3)	(4)	(5)	(6)	(7)
NEW YORK							
Albert Einstein Coll.	2.0	45/ 42	33/ 35	11/01	00/05	33/17	24/14
Australia United Hosp.	0.0	00/ 00	00/ 00	00/00	00/00	—/—	—/—
Children's Hos. (Buff.)	1.0	00/ 12	00/ 10	00/00	00/00	—/00	—/00
Columbia Presbyterian	2.2	00/ 00	00/ 00	00/00	00/00	—/—	—/—
Life Program	0.6	00/ 01	00/ 01	00/00	00/00	—/00	—/00
Long Island IVF	1.0	00/ 01	00/ 01	00/00	00/00	—/00	—/00
Mt. Sinai Hospital	1.5	12/ 14	12/ 08	04/01	00/02	33/38	33/21
NY Hospital-Cornell	2.0	30/ 31	30/ 24	04/03	00/02	13/24	13/16
SUNY-Syracuse	0.0	00/ 00	00/ 00	00/00	00/00	—/—	—/—
St. Luke's Roosevelt	3.0	01/ 02	01/ 02	00/00	00/00	00/00	00/00
U. of Rochester CARE	1.2	02/ 03	02/ 03	00/00	00/00	00/00	00/00
Wayne Decker IVF Program	0.0	00/ 00	00/ 00	00/00	00/00	—/—	—/—
NORTH CAROLINA							
Duke University Med.	4.0	10/ 11	09/ 07	01/01	00/00	11/14	10/09
NC Memorial Hospital	3.0	25/ NA	25/NA	03/NA	02/NA	20/NA	20/NA
N.C. Reprod. Center	0.0	00/ 00	00/ 00	00/00	00/00	—/—	—/—
OHIO							
Akron City Hospital	2.0	01/ 01	01/ 01	00/00	00/00	00/00	00/00
Bethesda Fertility	1.5	15/ 31	09/ 26	02/01	00/02	22/12	13/10

Cleveland Clinic Found.	2.6	02/ 00	02/ 00	01/00	00/00	50/—	50/—
Fertility Inst.-Cincinnati	3.0	46/ 38	46/ 38	06/05	00/02	13/18	13/18
Jewish Hosp. of Cin.	NA	18/ 15	15/ 07	00/00	00/00	00/00	00/00
MacDonald Hospital	4.0	00/ 00	00/ 00	00/00	00/00	—/—	—/—
Miami Valley Hospital	2.6	13/ 54	10/ 40	03/05	00/05	30/25	23/19
Midwest Reprod. Inst.	3.0	47/ 61	13/ 36	03/03	00/05	23/22	06/13
Mt. Sinai Med. Center	2.0	46/ 30	38/ 23	05/01	00/02	13/13	11/10
Ohio State	3.0	47/ 81	35/ 65	01/04	01/01	06/08	04/06
Riverside Reprod. Serv.	1.5	16/102	13/ 72	00/03	00/06	00/13	00/09
Univ. Reprod. Center	3.0	47/ 81	35/ 65	01/04	00/01	03/08	02/06
OKLAHOMA							
Henry Bennett Fertility	2.0	45/ 34	30/ 28	02/06	00/05	07/39	04/32
Hillcrest Fertility	2.3	00/ 00	00/ 00	00/00	00/00	—/—	—/—
OREGON							
Emanuel Hospital	1.3	02/ 02	02/ 02	00/00	00/00	00/00	00/00
Or. Health Science U.	2.3	32/ 28	16/ 18	02/03	00/05	13/44	06/29
PENNSYLVANIA							
Albert Einstein Med.	1.6	02/ 01	02/ 01	00/00	00/00	00/00	00/00
Christian Fert. Inst.-Easton	0.0	NA/NA	NA/NA	00/00	00/00	—/—	—/—
Endocrine Hist. Assoc.	0.0	00/ 00	00/ 00	00/00	00/00	—/—	—/—
Fert. Ctr. St. Lukes	3.0	00/ 79	59/ 52	03/06	00/05	05/21	—/14
Hospital of U. Penn.	3.2	18/ 32	16/ 27	00/03	00/01	00/15	00/13
Magee-Women's Hospital	2.0	62/108	40/ 69	00/08	00/21	00/42	00/27
Penn. Repro. Assoc.	3.7	166/162	130/120	29/08	00/25	22/27	17/20
Pittsburgh Institute	0.8	00/ 08	00/ 08	00/00	00/00	—/00	—/00
Women's Clinic Ltd.	0.0	00/ 00	00/ 00	00/00	00/00	—/—	—/—

GIFT DATA

PROGRAM	YEARS	87/88 STIM CYCLES	87/88 EGG RET	87/88 LIVE	87/88 CONT PREG	87/88 L+C/ER	87/88 L+C/SC
	(1)	(2)	(3)	(4)	(5)	(6)	(7)
RHODE ISLAND							
Womens & Infants Hosp.	0.0	00/ 00	00/ 00	00/00	00/00	—/—	—/—
SOUTH CAROLINA							
MUSC IVF Program	0.0	00/ 00	00/ 00	00/00	00/00	—/—	—/—
Southeastern Fertility	3.0	13/ 73	11/ 39	02/01	00/11	18/31	15/16
TENNESSEE							
E. Tenn. State Univ.	2.5	01/ 03	01/ 03	00/01	00/00	00/33	00/33
Pair (Memphis)	0.5	03/ 06	03/ 05	00/00	00/01	00/20	00/17
Univ. of Tenn. Knoxville	0.8	00/ 00	00/ 00	00/00	00/00	—/—	—/—
Vanderbilt Med. Centr.	3.0	33/ 16	25/ 14	01/04	00/02	04/43	03/38
TEXAS							
Baylor GIFT/IVF	3.0	NA/NA	23/ 18	02/01	00/03	09/22	NA/NA
Center for Repro. Med.	2.3	26/ 10	23/ 09	00/02	02/01	09/33	08/30
Ft. Worth Infert. Ctr.	2.3	05/ 07	05/ 07	00/01	00/01	00/29	00/29
Houston Reproductive	4.0	04/ 01	04/ 01	00/00	00/00	00/00	00/00
J. B. Belue, M.D.	2.2	20/ 12	13/ 07	02/01	00/00	15/14	10/08
OB & GYN Associates	4.0	125/104	102/ 91	22/07	00/08	22/16	18/14
Presb. Hosp. Dallas	3.4	50/ 49	31/ 24	11/02	00/06	35/33	22/16
Scott & White Clinic	0.4	00/ 03	00/ 02	00/00	00/01	—/50	—/33

Trinity IVF-ET Program	4.0	04/ 12	04/ 12	00/03	00/01	00/33	00/33
St. David's-Austin	3.0	82/ 06	59/ 04	06/00	00/00	10/00	07/00
U of Tx-SW Med School	2.0	07/ 02	07/ 02	00/00	00/00	00/00	00/00
U of Tx-Galveston	2.0	03/ 12	03/ 12	01/02	00/01	33/25	33/25
UTAH							
University of Utah	2.6	18/ 09	13/ 08	04/02	00/01	05/38	22/33
VERMONT							
University of Vermont	2.7	01/ 00	01/ 00	00/00	00/00	00/—	00/—
VIRGINIA							
Henrico Drs. Hosp.	2.9	12/ 17	11/ 16	03/01	00/04	27/31	25/29
Jones Institute	3.0	01/ 02	01/ 02	00/00	00/01	00/50	00/50
Medical College of Va.	0.3	00/ 01	00/ 01	00/00	00/00	—/00	—/00
University of Va.	0.5	04/ 10	04/ 06	00/00	00/02	00/33	00/20
WASHINGTON							
Fert Clin Puget Sound	4.0	111/26	103/26	00/00	00/08	00/31	00/31
Rice & Associates	0.3	00/02	00/02	00/00	00/02	—/100	00/100
Seattle Fert & GYN	3.4	141/57	96/47	27/10	00/11	28/45	19/37
Seattle Women's Clinic	1.9	06/ 06	04/ 04	01/01	00/00	25/25	17/17
Swedish Hosp. Med. Cen.	3.4	204/101	137/ 75	34/13	00/14	25/36	17/27
Univ. of Washington	2.0	10/ 06	07/ 05	00/03	00/02	00/100	00/83
WEST VIRGINIA							
W. Virginia Univ.	1.0	00/ 50	00/ 35	00/05	00/04	—/26	—/18

GIFT DATA

PROGRAM	YEARS	87/88 STIM CYCLES	87/88 EGG RET	87/88 LIVE	87/88 CONT PREG	87/88 L+C/ER	87/88 L+C/SC
	(1)	(2)	(3)	(4)	(5)	(6)	(7)
WISCONSIN							
Advanced Institute of Fert.	4.0	NA/NA	29/ 33	04/04	00/00	14/12	NA/NA
Appleton Family Fert.	1.2	01/ 12	01/ 12	00/01	00/03	00/33	00/33
Univ. of Wisconsin	1.0	00/ 01	00/ 01	00/00	00/00	—/00	—/00

appendix two

Resources

SOURCES OF INFORMATION

General Information

The American Fertility Society (AFS)
2140 11th Avenue South/Suite 200
Birmingham, AL 35205-2800
(205) 251-9764

American College of Obstetricians and Gynecologists (ACOG)
600 Maryland Avenue, S.W./Suite 300
Washington, D.C. 20024
(202) 638-5577

SERONO SYMPOSIA, U.S.A.
100 Longwater Circle
Norwell, MA 02061
(617) 982-9000
(800) 283-8088

Congressional Subcommittee Report

Subcommittee on Regulation, Business Opportunities, and Energy
Room B363 RHOB
Washington, D.C. 20515

Information on Surrogate Parenting

ICNY
14 East 60th Street/ Suite 1204
New York, N.Y. 10022
(212) 371-0811

Center for Surrogate Parenting, Inc.
8383 Wilshire Boulevard/Suite 750
Beverly Hills, California 90211
(213) 655-1974

Adoption

Child Welfare League of America
67 Irving Place
New York, N.Y. 10003

North American Council on Adoptable Children (NACAG)
1346 Connecticut Avenue, S.W./Suite 229
Washington, D.C. 20036
1821 University Avenue
St. Paul, MN 55104
(612) 644-3036

SUPPORT GROUP

RESOLVE, Inc.
National Office
5 Water Street
Arlington, MA 02174
(617) 643-2424

IVF PROGRAMS REPORTING TO THE CONGRESSIONAL SURVEY

NOTE: There are some discrepancies in addresses and telephone numbers in different parts of the congressioal report. We have attempted to provide the information as correctly as possible, but some errors may exist. In addition, the survey report listed some programs for which we could not find data. We listed these addresses and noted that no data were available or there was no activity reported.

ALABAMA

(Assisted Reproductive)
Assisted Reproductive Technology
(ART) Program
2006 Brookwood Medical Center Drive/
#508
Birmingham, AL 35209
(205) 870-9784

(Univ. of Al.-Birmingham)
University of Alabama Birmingham
IVF/GIFT Program
Department of Ob/Gyn
547 Old Hillman Building
University Station
Birmingham, AL 35294
(205) 934-7121

(Univ. of South Alabama)
University of South Alabama
IVF/GIFT Program: Dept. of Ob/Gyn
CC/CB
Division of Reproductive Endocrinology
Mobile, AL 36688
(205) 460-7173

ARIZONA

(Az. Cent. Fert. Studies)
Arizona Center for Fertility Studies
IVF-ET Program
4614 East Shea Blvd., D-250
Phoenix, AZ 85028
(602) 996-7896

(Az. Fertility Institute)
Arizona Fertility Institute
2850 N. 24th Street/Suite 500-A
Phoenix, AZ 85008
(602) 468-3840

(Az. Repro. Inst. of Tucson)
The Reproductive Institute of
Tucson
Building G Suite 7
1200 North El Dorado Place
Tucson, AZ 85715
(602) 290-8818

(Southwest Fertility)
Southwest Fertility Center
3125 North 32nd St. Suite 200
Phoenix, AZ 85018
(602) 956-7481

CALIFORNIA

(Alta Bates Hospital)
Alta Bates Hospital
In Vitro Fertilization Program
3001 Colby Street
Berkeley, CA 94705
(415) 540-1416

(AMI South Bay Hospital)
AMI-South Bay Hospital
In Vitro Fertilization Center
514 South Prospect Avenue
Redondo Beach, CA 90277
(213) 318-4741

(Cal.-Irvine IVF-GIFT)
UC Irvine/Memorial Women's Hos-
pital IVF/GIFT Program
2880 Atlantic Avenue Suite 220
Long Beach, CA 90806
(213) 595-2229

(Cedars-Sinai Med Center)
Cedars-Sinai Hospital
Center for Reproductive Medicine
444 South San Vicente Blvd. 11th Floor
Los Angeles, CA 90048

(Central Ca. IVF Program)
Central California IVF Program
Fresno Community Hospital
PO Box 1232
Fresno, CA 93715
(209) 439-1914

(Century City Hosp.)
Century City Hospital
IVF Program
2070 Century Park East
Los Angeles, CA 90067
(213) 201-6619

(Fert & Repro Health)
Fertility & Reproductive Health Institute of Northern California
2516 Samaritan Drive Suita A
San Jose, CA 95124

(Forest Fertility Center)
Forest Fertility Center
2110 Forest Avenue
San Jose, CA 95128
(408) 288-9933

(Hoag Fertility Service)
Hoaf Fertility Services
Hoag Memorial Hospital
351 Hospital Road Suite 316
Newport, CA 92663
(714) 760-2395

(Hosp of Good Sam.)
Hospital of Good Samaritan
Institute for Reproductive Medicine
1245 Wilshire Blvd. Suite 905
Los Angeles, CA 90017
(213) 482-4552

(Huntington Repro. Ctr.)
Huntington Reproductive Center
39 Congress Street, Suite 202
Pasadena, CA 91105
(818) 440-9161

(Infertil Med Group-San Diego)
Infertility, Gynecology & Obstetrics Medical Group
9330 Genessee Ave. Suite 220
San Diego, CA 92121
(619) 455-7520

(John Muir Memorial)
John Muir Memorial Hospital
Dept. of Ob/Gyn: IVF Program
1601 Ygnacio Valley Road
Walnut Creet, CA 94598
(415) 947-5285

(North. Calif. Fert.)
Northern California Fertility Center
87 Scripps Drive/Suite 202
Sacramento, CA 95825
(916) 929-3596

(Northridge Hosp.)
Northridge Hospital Medical Center
IVF Program
18300 Roscoe Blvd.
Northridge, CA 91328
(818) 885-5420

(Nova Fertility Center)
Nova Fertility Center
101 S. San Mateo Drive #201
San Mateo, California
(415) 340-0500

(Pacific Fertility Cen.)
Pacific Fertility Center
2100 Webster Street/Suite 220
San Francisco, CA 94115
(415) 923-3344

Scripps Clinic Fertility Center
10666 North Torrey Pines Road
La Jolla, CA 92037

(S. Cal. Fertility Ins.)
Southern California Fertility Center
California Institute for IVF
Right to Parenthood Program
12301 Wilshire Blvd. Suite 415
Los Angeles, CA 90025
(213) 820-3723

(Stanford University)
Reproductive Endocrinology & Infertility Clinic
Stanford University
Dept. of Ob/Gyn
S-385 Medical Center
Stanford, CA 94305
(415) 723-5251

(UCLA Medical Center)
UCLA School of Medicine
Department of Ob/Gyn: IVF Program
CHS-22-168
Los Angeles, CA 90024
(213) 825-7755

(UCSF Fertility Assoc.)
UCSF Fertility Associates
University of California San Francisco
Dept. of Ob/Gyn & Reproductive Sciences
Box 0132 Rm. M-1489
San Francisco, CA 94143
(415) 476-2224

(USC School of Med.)
USC School of Medicine
California Reproductive Health Institute
1338 South Hope Street
Los Angeles, CA 90015
(213) 742-5970

(Whittier Hospital)
Whittier Hospital Medical Center
The Genesis Program for IVF
Center Human Development
15151 Janine Drive
Whittier, CA 90605
(213) 945-3561 ext. 555

COLORADO

(Inf/Gyn/Obs-Englewood)
Infertility, Gynecology & Obstetrics
601 E. Hampden #185
Englewood, CO 80110
(303) 788-6371

(Reproductive Genetics)
Conceptions Unlimited
455 S. Hudson Street, Level Three
Denver, CO 80222
(303) 399-1464

CONNECTICUT

(Mt. Sinai Hospital)
Mount Sinai Hospital
Department of Ob/Gyn
Divisionof Reproductive Endocrinology
and Infertility
675 Tower Avenue
Hartford, CT 06112
(203) 242-6201

(UCONN School of Med.)
**Reproductive Endocrinology &
Fertility**
University of Connecticut Health Center
Department of Ob/Gyn
263 Farmington Avenue
Farmington, CT 06732
(203) 679-4580

(Yale School of Med.)
Yale University Medical School
Department of Ob/Gyn: IVF Program
333 Cedar Street
New Haven, CT 06510
(203) 785-4019

DELAWARE

(Repro. Endo and Fert.-Newark)
**Reproductive Endocrine and Fertil-
ity Center**
Medical Center of Delaware
4745 Ogletown-Stanton Road
Newark, DE 19718
(302) 738-4600

DISTRICT OF COLUMBIA

(Columbia Hos. for Wom.)
**Columbia Hospital for Women Med-
ical Center**
IVF Program
2440 M. Street, NW/Suite 401
Washington, DC 20034
(202) 293-5249

226 New Options in Fertility

(GW University IVF)
George Washington University Medical Center
Department of Ob/Gyn: IVF Program
2150 Pennsylvania Avenue, NW
Washington, DC 20037
(202) 994-4614

FLORIDA

(Fert Cen of Boca Raton)
Fertility Institute of Boca Raton
West Boca Medical Center
21644 State Road 7, Highway 441
Boca Raton, FL 33428
(407) 488-8000

(Florida Fertility)
Florida Fertility Institute
3451 66th North
St. Petersburg, FL 33710
(813) 384-4000

(Humana Women's Hosp.)
Humana Women's Hospital
University of South Florida
3030 West Buffalo Avenue
Tampa, FL 33606
(813) 872-2988

(Jacksonville Mem. Med.)
Memorial Medical Center of Jacksonville
In Vitro Fertilization Program
3343 University Boulevard South
Jacksonville, FL 32216
(904) 391-1149

(N.W. Fla. Gulf Breeze)
The Fertility Institute of Northwest Florida, Inc.
Gulf Breeze Hospital, Suite 202
Gulf Breeze, FL 32561
(904) 934-3900

(NW Center for Infert.)
Northwest Center for Infertility & Reproductive Endocrinology
5800 Colonial Drive, Suite 200
Margate, FL 33063
(305) 972-5001

(Park Ave. Womens Centr.)
Park Avenue Women's Center
University of Florida Associates
817 NW 56 Terrace, Suite C
Gainesville, FL 32605
(904) 392-6200

(Sand Lake IVF Center.)
Sand Lake Hospital
Center for Infertility and Reproductive Medicine, Orlando
9430 Turkey Lake Road, Suite 218
Orlando, FL 32819
(407) 843-0587

(University of Miami)
University of Miami
Department of Ob/Gyn
P.O. Box 016960
Miami, FL 33101
(305) 547-5818

GEORGIA

(Augusta Reprod. Bio.)
Augusta Reproductive Biology Associates
University Hospital
810-812 Chafee Avenue
Augusta, GA 30904
(404) 724-0228

(Med. College of Ga.)
Medical College of Georgia
Humana Hospital-IVF Section
Dept. of Ob-Gyn Ck-147
Augusta, GA 30912
(404) 721-3832

(Reproductive Biology)
Reproductive Biology Associates
993-D Johnson Ferry Road/Suite 330
Atlanta, GA 30342
(404) 843-3064

HAWAII

(Kauai Med. Group)
Kauai Medical Group
University of Hawaii
Wilcox Memorial Hospital
Department of Ob/Gyn
3420-B Kuhio Highway
Lihue, HI 96766
(808) 245-1571

(Pacific IVF Institute)
Pacific In Virto Fertilization Institute
Kapiolani Hospital
1319 Punahou Street, Suite 1040
Honolulu, HI 96826
(808) 946-2226

ILLINOIS

(Evanston and Glenbrook)
The Evanston and Glenbrook Hospitals
IVF Program
2050 Pfingsten Road, Suite 350
Glenview, IL 60025
(312) 729-6450

(Masonic Medical Cent.)
Illinois Masonic Medical Center
IVF Illinois
Fifth Floor, Center Court
836 Wellington
Chicago, IL 60657
(312) 883-7096

(Michael Reese Hospital)
Michael Reese Hospital & Medical Center
IVF-ET Program
31st Street at Lake Shore Drive

Chicago, IL 60616
(312) 791-4000

(Northwestern Memorial)
Northwestern Memorial Hospital
IVF Program
Prentice Womens Hospital
333 East Superior Street, Suite 454
Chicago, IL 60612
(312) 908-1364

(Rush Presb-St. Luke's)
IVF Program
Rush Presbyterian-St. Luke's Medical Center
1653 West Congress Parkway
Chicago, IL 60612
(312) 942-6609

(Mt. Sinai-Chicago)
Mount Sinai Hospital Medical Center
Department of Ob/Gyn: IVF Program
California Avenue at 15th Street
Chicago, IL 60608
(312) 650-6727

(Un. of Illinois Med. Cen.)
University of Illinois College of Medicine
Department of Ob/Gyn M/C 808
840 South Wood Street
Chicago, IL 60612
(312) 996-7388

INDIANA

(Center for Reprod.)
Center for Reproduction & Transplantation Immunology
Methodist Hospital of Indiana
1701 N. Senate Blvd.
Indianapolis, IN 46202
(317) 929-5950

(Indiana University)
Indiana University Medical Center
Department of Ob/Gyn-Reproductive Endocrinology

926 West Michigan Street, N-262
Indianapolis, IN 46223
(317) 274-4037

(Pregnancy Initiation)
Pregnancy Initiation Center
Humana Womens Hospital
8091 Township Line Road, Suite 110
Indianapolis, IN 46260
(317) 876-0539

IOWA

(University of Iowa)
University of Iowa Hospitals and
Clinics
Center for Advanced Reproductive Care
Iowa City, IA 52242
(319) 356-8483

KANSAS

(Reprod. Resource Cen.)
Reproductive Resource Center of
Greater Kansas City
10600 Quivera, Suite 110
Overland Park, KS 66215
(913) 894-2323

(Univ. Kansas Wichita)
University of Kansas School of
Medicine:
Wichita Center for Reproductive
Medicine
HCA-Wesley Medical Center
Division of Reproductive Endocrinology
2903 East Central
Wichita, KS 67214-4976
(316) 687-2112

University of Kansas College of
Health Sciences
Ob/Gyn Foundation
39th and Rainbow Blvd.
Kansas City, KS 66103

KENTUCKY

(Fertility Institute)
Fertility Institute
Plunkett & Thompson, M.D.'s
40 N. Grand Avenue, Suite 302
Ft. Thomas, KY 41075

(Norton Hospital)
Infertility Program
Norton Hospital
University of Louisville
200 E. Chestnut St.
P.O. Box 35070
Louisville, KY 40202-5070
(502) 562-8154

(University of Kentucky)
University of Kentucky
Department of Ob/Gyn
800 Rose St.
Kentucky Center for Reproductive Medicine
Lexington, KY 40536
(606) 233-5410

LOUISIANA

(Fertility Center-Kenner)
Fertility Center of Louisiana
200 West Esplanade Avenue/Suite 210
Kenner, LA 70065
(504) 464-8622

(Fertility Inst. New Orleans)
The Fertility Institute of New
Orleans
Humana Womens Hospital
6020 Bullard Avenue
New Orleans, LA 70128
(504) 246-8971

MARYLAND

(Ctr. for Reprod. Studies-Balt.)
Union Memorial Hospital
Center for Reproductive Studies and
Infertility

201 East University Parkway
Baltimore, MD 21218
(301) 554-2942

(Johns Hopkins)
The Johns Hopkins Hospital
Division of Reproductive Endocrinology
600 North Wolfe Street
Baltimore, MD 21205
(301) 955-2016

(Montgomery Inf. Inst.)
Montgomery Fertility Institute
10215 Fernwood Road #303-304
Bethesda, MD 20817
(301) 897-8850

(University of Maryland)
University of Maryland-Baltimore
Ob/Gyn Associates
419 West Redwood Street, Rm. 500
Baltimore, MD 21209
(301) 328-2304

(Women's Hosp. Center)
Women's Hospital Fertility Center:
  IVF Program
Greater Baltimore Medical Center
6701 North Charles Street
Baltimore, MD 21204
(301) 828-2484

MASSACHUSETTS

(Atlanticare Fertility)
Atlanticare Fertility Center
500 Lynnfield Street
Lynn, MA 01904
(617) 581-0330

(Beth Israel-Boston)
Beth Israel Hospital
IVF/GIFT Program
330 Brookline Avenue
Boston, MA 02215
(617) 735-5923

(Boston IVF)
Boston IVF
1 Brookline Place, Suite 602
Brookline, MA 02146
(617) 735-9000 x202

(Brigham & Women's Hosp.)
Brigham and Women's Hospital
IVF Program
75 Francis Street
Boston, MA 02115
(617) 732-5444

(New England Med. Centr.)
Neew England Medical Center Hos-
  pitals
Department of Ob/Gyn-IVF Clinic
750 Washington Street, Box 36
Boston, MA 02111
(617) 956-6049

(No activity)
IVF Australia-Boston
Waltham/Weston Hospital & Medical
  Center
20 Hope Avenue
Waltham, MA 02254-9116
(800) 288-4832
(617) 647-6263

MICHIGAN

(Blodgett Memorial IFV)
Blodgett Memorial Medical Center
IVF Program
1900 Wealthy Street SE, Suite 330
Grand Rapids, MI 49506
(616) 774-0700

(Hutzel Hosp./Wayne St.)
Hutzel Hospital
Wayne State University: IVF Program
4707 St. Antoine
Detroit, MI 48201
(313) 745-7693

(Oakwood Hospital)
Oakwood Hospital
Center for Reproductive Medicine
18181 Oakwood Blvd., Suite 100G
Dearborn, MI 48124
(313) 593-5880

(Schi Reprod. Endo.)
SCHI Reproductive Endocrinology
Saginaw General Hospital
1000 Houghton Avenue
Saginaw, MI 48602
(517) 771-6838

(Univ. Mi. Med. Centr.)
**University of Michigan Medical
Center**
Division of Reproductive Endocrinology
& Infertility
L2021 Womens Hospital-D2202 MOB
Box 0718
Ann Arbor, MI 48109-0718
(313) 936-7401

(William Beaumont Hosp.)
William Beaumont Hospital
IVF Program
3601 West 13 Mile Road
Royal Oak, MI 48072
(313) 288-7937

MINNESOTA

(U. of Minnesota)
Women's Health Center
University of Minnesota VIP Program
Department of Ob/Gyn
Box 395, Mayo Memorial Building
420 Delaware Street, SE
Minneapolis, MN 55455
(612) 626-3232

MISSISSIPPI

(U. Miss. Med. Center)
**University of Mississippi Medical
Center**
IVF Program
Department of Ob/Gyn

2500 N. State Street
Jackson, MS 39216
(601) 984-5330

MISSOURI

(Washington U. Jewish)
Jewish Hospital at Washington University Medical Center
Department of Ob/Gyn
216 South Kingshighway
St. Louis, MO 63110
(314) 454-7834

NEBRASKA

(Methodist Hospital)
Nebraska Methodist Hospital
Department of Ob/Gyn
8303 Dodge Street
Omaha, NE 68114
(402) 390-4138

(University of Nebraska)
**University of Nebraska Medical
Center**
Department of Ob/Gyn
42nd and Dewey Avenue
Omaha, NE 68144
(402) 559-6151

NEVADA

(Northern Nv. Fertility)
Northern Nevada Fertility Institute
350 West Sixth Street, Suite 3AB
Reno, NV 89503
(702) 688-5600

NEW HAMPSHIRE

(Dartmouth-Hitchcock)
**Dartmouth-Hitchcock Medical
Center**
2 Maynard Street, Clinic 500
Hanover, NH 03756
(603) 646-8255

NEW JERSEY

(Robert Wood Johnson)
UMDNJ-Robert Wood Johnson Medical School
IVF Program: Department of Ob/Gyn
#1 Robert Wood Johnson Place, CN19
New Brunswick, NJ 08903
(201) 937-7716

(UMDNJ NJ Med Schools)
UMDNJ-New Jersey Medical School, Newark
Center for Reproductive Medicine F342
150 Bergen Street
Newark, NJ 07103
(201) 456-6029

NEW MEXICO

(Presbyterian IVF)
Presbyterian Hospital
IVF Program
201 Cedar Street Southeast/#307
Albuquerque, NM 87106
(505) 247-3333

NEW YORK

(Albert Einstein Coll.)
Albert Einstein College of Medicine
Fertility and Hormone Center
88 Ashford Avenue
Dobbs Ferry, NY 10522
(914) 693-8820

(Australia United Hosp.)
IVF Australia at United Hospital
406 Boston Post Road
Port Chester, NY 10573
(914) 934-7481

[Children's Hos. (Buff.)]
Children's Hospital of Buffalo
Reproductive Endocrinology Unit
140 Hodge Avenue
Buffalo, NY 14222
(716) 878-7698

(Columbia Presbyterian)
Columbia-Presbyterian Medical Center
Presbyterian Hospital IVF Program
622 West 168th Street PH-16 IVF Office
New York, NY 10032
(212) 305-9921

(Life Program)
Life Program
Albany Memorial Hospital
600 Northern Blvd.
Albany, NY 12204
(518) 482-1007

(Long Island IVF)
Long Island IVF
60 North Country Road
Port Jefferson, NY 11777
(516) 331-7575

(Mt. Sinai Hospital)
Mount Sinai Medical Center
IVF Program
1212 5th Avenue Box 1175
New York, NY 10029
(212) 241-5927

(NY Hospital-Cornell)
Cornell University Medical Center
Program for In Vitro Fertilization
Center for Reproductive Medicine and Infertility
525 East 68th Street/Box 1
New York, NY 10021
(212) 746-1762

(SUNY-Syracuse)
SUNY Health Science Center
Crouse Irving Memorial Hospital
Department of Ob/Gyn
Division of Reproductive Endocrinology
Syracuse, NY 13210
(315) 749-7905

(St. Luke's Roosevelt)
St. Luke's Roosevelt Hospital Center
IVF-ET Program
1111 Amsterdam Avenue
New York, NY 10025
(212) 523-3459

(U. of Rochester CARE)
University of Rochester Care Program
University of Rochester Medical Center
601 Elmwood Avenue/Box 668
Rochester, NY 14618
(716) 275-5747

(Wayne Decker IVF Program)
Wayne H. Decker IVF Program
1430 Second Avenue, Suite 103
New York, NY 10021
(212) 744-5500

NORTH CAROLINA

(Duke University Med.)
Duke University Medical Center
Department of Ob/Gyn Box 3527
Durham, NC 27710
(919) 684-5327

(NC Memorial Hospital)
UNC Medical School
In Vitro Fertilization-GIFT Program
The North Carolina Memorial Hospital
Department of Ob/Gyn Box 7570
Chapel Hill, NC 27599-7570
(919) 966-1150

(N.C. Reprod. Center)
North Carolina Reproductive Center
P.O. Box 4052
1200 N. Elm Street
Greensboro, NC 27404
(919) 373-8555

(Satellite of UNC, Chapel Hill)
Women's Specialty Center
Charlotte Memorial Hospital
1901 Brunswick Avenue
Charlotte, NC 28207

OHIO

(Akron City Hospital)
Akron City Hospital
IVF Program
525 East Market Street
Akron, OH 44309
(216) 375-3585

(Bethesda Fertility)
Bethesda Fertility Center
619 Oak Street, 3 South
Cincinnati, OH 45206
(513) 569-6433

(No activity)
Center for Reproductive Health
University of Cincinnati School of Medicine
Bethesda & Eden Avenue (ML 456)
Cincinnati, OH 45267
(513) 558-8440

(Cleveland Clinic Found.)
Cleveland Clinic Foundation
IVF Program
9500 Euclid Avenue
Cleveland, OH 44195-5037
(216) 444-2240

(Fertility Inst.-Cincinnati)
2800 Winslow/Suite 203
Cincinnati, OH 45206
(513) 441-1201

(Jewish Hosp. of Cin.)
Jewish Hospital of Cincinnati
Department of Ob/Gyn
3200 Burnet Avenue
Cincinnati, OH 45229
(513) 221-3062

(MacDonald Hospital)
MacDonald Hospital for Women
2105 Abington Road/Suite 1632
Cleveland, OH 44106
(216) 844-1514

(Miami Valley Hospital)
Miami Valley Hospital
Fertility Program
1 Wyoming Street
Dayton, OH 45409
(513) 228-1510

(Midwest Reprod. Inst.)
Midwest Reproductive Institute
c/o Nichols Vorys, MD
1492 E. Broad St. Suite 1203
Columbus, OH 43205
(614) 253-0003

(Mt. Sinai Med. Center)
Mount Sinai Medical Center
Laboratory for In Vitro Fertilization &
  Embryo Transfer
1 Mount Sinai Drive
Cleveland, OH 44106
(216) 421-5884

(Ohio State University)
University Reproductive Center
1654 Upham Drive, MH-535
Columbus, OH 43210
(614) 293-8511

(Riverside Reprod. Serv.)
Univ. Reprod. Center
Riverside Reproductive Services
3726 K Olentangy River Road
Columbus, OH 43214
(614) 261-5032

OKLAHOMA

(Henry Bennett Fertility)
Henry G. Bennett Fertility Institute
3433 NW 56th Street, Suite 200
Oklahoma City, OK 73112
(405) 949-6060

(Hillcrest Fertility)
Hillcrest Fertility Center
1145 South Utica, Suite 1209
Tulsa, OK 74104
(918) 584-2870

OREGON

(Emanuel Hospital)
Northwest Fertility Center
Emanuel Hospital
2801 North Gantenbain Avenue
Portland, Oregon 97227
(503) 280-3097

(Or. Health Science U.)
Oregon Health Sciences University
Reproductive Research & Fertility Program
3181 SW Sam Jackson Park Road L466
Portland, OR 97201
(503) 279-8449

PENNSYLVANIA

(Albert Einstein Med.)
Albert Einstein Medical Center
Department of Ob/Gyn Klein POB-400
York and Tabor Roads
Philadelphia, PA 19141
(215) 456-7990

(Christian Fert Inst.-Easton)
Christian Fertility Institute
241 North 13th Steet
Easton, PA 18042
(215) 250-9700

(Endocrine Hist. Assoc.)
Endocrine Histology Associates
7447 Old York Road
Melrose Park, PA 19126
(215) 635-5518

(Fert. Ctr. St. Lukes)
Fertility Center at St. Lukes Hospital
821 Ostrum Street
Bethlehem, PA 18015
(215) 691-4825

(Hospital of U. Penn.)
Hospital of the University of Penn-
  sylvania
Department of Ob/Gyn-One Dulles
Building

3400 Spruce Street, Suite 106
Philadelphia, PA 19104
(215) 662-6560

(Magee-Women's Hospital)
Program for IVF and Embryo Transfer
Magee Women's Hospital
Department of Ob/Gyn
Pittsburgh, PA 15213
(412) 647-1670

(Penn. Repro. Assoc.)
Pennsylvania Reproductive Associates at Pennsylvania Hospital
829 Spruce Street
Philadelphia, PA 19107
(215) 829-5095

(Pittsburgh Institute)
Pittsburgh Institute of Reproductive Medicine
510 South Aiken Avenue/Suite 312
Pittsburgh, PA 15232
(412) 622-1720

(Women's Clinic LTD.)
Women's Clinic LTD
301 South Seventh Avenue Suite 240
West Reading, PA 19611
(215) 378-1348

RHODE ISLAND

(Women's & Infants Hosp.)
Women's and Infant's Hospital of Rhode Island
161 Dudley Street
Providence, RI 02905
(401) 274-1100 ext. 1564

SOUTH CAROLINA

(MUSC IVF Program)
Medical University of South Carolina (MUSC)
Department of Ob/Gyn
171 Ashley Avenue

Charleston, SC 29425
(803) 972-8351

(Southeastern Fertility)
The Southeastern Fertility Center
900 Bowman Road, Suite 108
Mount Pleasant, SC 29464
(803) 881-3900

TENNESSEE

(E. Tenn. State Univ.)
East Tennessee State University College of Medicine
Department of Ob/Gyn
Box 19570A
Johnson City, TN 37614
(615) 929-6659

[Pair (Memphis)]
University of Tennessee-Memphis
Program for Advanced Infertility & Reproduction
66 North Pauline
Memphis, TN 38105
(901) 528-6634

(Univ. of Tenn. Knoxville)
University of Tennessee Fertility Center
1924 Alcoa Highway, U-27
Knoxville, Tn 37920
(615) 544-9305

(Vanderbilt Med. Centr.)
Vanderbilt University
Center for Fertility and Reproductive Research
IVF Program
D-3200 Medical Center North
Nashville, TN 37232
(615) 322-6576

(Data not reported in survey format)
East Tennessee Baptist Hospital
Family Life Center
7A Office 715

Blount Avenue, Box 1788
Knoxville, Tn 37901
(615) 573-0031

TEXAS

(Baylor GIFT/IVF)
Baylor College of Medicine
Department of Ob/Gyn
#1 Baylor Medical Plaza
Houston, TX 77054
(713) 798-7500 ext. 277

(Center for Repro. Med.)
Center for Reproductive Medicine
8100 Fredericksberg Road
San Antonio, TX 78229
(512) 567-4938

(Ft. Worth Infert. Ctr.)
Fort Worth Infertility Center
1325 Pennsylvania Avenue, Suite 750
Fort Worth, TX 76104
(817) 335-0909

(Houston Reproductive)
Houston Reproductive Center
Sam Houston Memorial Hospital
1615 Hillendahl Boulevard
Houston, TX 77055
(713) 932-5679

(J.B. Belue, M.D.)
J.B. Belue, M.D.
120 E. Charnwood
Tyler, TX 75701
(214) 597-8371

(OB & GYN Associates)
Ob & Gyn Associates
7550 Fannin
Houston, TX 77054
(713) 797-9123

(Presb. Hosp. Dallas)
Presbyterian Hospital of Dallas
8160 Walnut Hill Lane/Suite 320
PO Box 17

Dallas, TX 75231
(214) 363-6322

(Scott & White Clinic)
Scott & White Clinic
Texas A & M College of Medicine
2401 South 31st Street
Temple, TX 76508
(817) 774-3321

(St. Davids-Austin)
Saint David's Community Hospital
IVF-GIFT Program
1302 West 38th Street
PO Box 4039
Austin, TX 78765
(512) 397-4127

(Trinity IVF-ET Program)
Trinity IVF/ET Program
Trinity Medical Center
4333 North Josey Lane, Suite 200
Carrolton, TX 75010
(214) 394-0114

(U of Tx-SW Med School)
University of Texas SW Medical
School
Division of Reproductive Endocrinology
Department of Ob/Gyn
5323 Harry Hines Boulevard
Dallas, TX 75235
(214) 688-3791

(U. of Tx-Galveston)
University of Texas Medical Branch
IVF Program
Department of Ob/Gyn
Galveston, TX 77550
(409) 761-3985

(No data reported)
Texas Fertility Center
HCA Medical Plaza, 4th Floor
1612 West Humbolt
Ft. Worth, TX 76104
(817) 336-GIFT

(No data reported)
University of Texas Health Science Center
Department of Reproductive Science
6431 Fannin, Suite 3.204
Houston, TX 77030

(No data reported)
Texas Tech University Health Sciences Center
Department of Ob/Gyn
3601 4th Street
Lubbock, TX 79430

UTAH

(University of Utah)
University of Utah
Department of Ob/Gyn
Fertility Center Office
50 Medical Drive North
Salt Lake City, UT 84132
(801) 581-4837

VERMONT

(University of Vermont)
University of Vermont College of Medicine
Division of Reproductive Endocrinology
Department of Ob/Gyn
Burlington, VT 05405
(802) 656-2272

VIRGINIA

(Henrico Drs. Hosp.)
Henrico Doctors Hospital
Richmond Center for Fertility and Endocrinology
7605 Forest Avenue, Suite 207
Richmond, VA 23229
(804) 285-9700

(Jones Institute)
Jones Institute for Reproductive Medicine
Eastern Virginia Medical School
Hofheimer Hall, Sixth Floor

825 Fairfax Avenue
Norfolk, VA 23507
(804) 446-8948

(Medical College of Va.)
Medical College of Virginia
IVF Program
Box 34, MCV Station
Richmond, VA 23298
(804) 786-9638

(University of Va.)
University of Virginia Health Sciences Center
IVF/GIFT Program
Division of Reproductive Endocrinology
Box 387
Charlottesville, VA 22908
(804) 924-0312

WASHINGTON

(Fert Clin Puget Sound)
Fertility Clinic of Puget Sound
South 36th and Pacific Avenue
Tacoma, WA 98304
(206) 475-5433

(Rice & Associates)
Rice and Associates
Fifth & Browne Med. Center West/Suite 410
Spokane, WA 99203
(509) 455-8111

(Seattle Fert & GYN)
Seattle Fertility & Gynecology
1229 Madison, Suite 1220
Seattle, WA 98104
(206) 682-9935

(Seattle Women's Clinic)
Seattle Women's Clinic
IVF Program
801 Broadway, Suite 511
Seattle, WA 98112
(206) 292-2200

(Swedish Hosp. Med. Cen.)
Swedish Hospital Medical Center
Reproductive Genetics Laboratory
747 Summit Avenue
Seattle, WA 98104
(206) 386-2483

(Univ. of Washington)
University of Washington
Special Fertility Programs
Department of Ob/Gyn RH20
University Hospital
Seattle, WA 98195
(206) 548-4071

WEST VIRGINIA

(W. Virginia Univ.)
West Virginia University
Department of Ob/Gyn
830 Pennsylvania Avenue/Suite 304
Charleston, WV 25302
(304) 342-0816

WISCONSIN

(Advanced Inst. of Fertility)
Advanced Institute of Fertility
2000 West Kilbourn Avenue, Suite 462
Milwaukee, WI 53233
(414) 937-5437

(Appleton Family Fert.)
Appleton Medical Center
Family Fertility Program
1818 North Meade Street
Appleton, WI 54911
(414) 739-0114

(Univ. of Wisconsin)
University of Wisconsin Clinics
Madison Infertility Clinic
600 Highland Avenue
H4/630 CSC
Madison, WI 53792
(608) 263-1217

(Division of Advanced Institute of Fert.)
Waukesha Memorial Hospital
IVF Program
765 American Avenue
Waukesha, WI 53186
(414) 544-2722

Twenty
Questions For
Information At
A Glance

Manufacturers of high-tech electronic products such as sophisticated stereo equipment often provide a section in their instructions designed for consumers who want to plug it in and enjoy the music before reading in detail about how many decibels are required to blow out their eardrums. The purpose of this appendix is similar. The answers to the following twenty questions will give you a basic working knowledge of assisted reproductive procedures, but without the details. However, if you are considering entering a program or are in the midst of conventional infertility treatment, this chapter is *not enough* to help you make informed choices and to know if accepted procedures are being followed. You may want to start here, but we urge you to read the entire book to obtain all the information you will need.

1. What is assisted reproduction? Assisted reproductive technology (ART) consists of procedures beyond conventional infertility treatment. They have as their common characteristic the technical manipulation of the sperm and the egg outside the body for their replacement into the reproductive organs to achieve a pregnancy. They may be replaced as eggs and sperm or early embryos. They can be placed into the woman's uterus or fallopian tube.

2. What procedures are considered to be ART? Currently the clinically available procedures include:

- IVF (In Vitro Fertilization) The most advanced procedure in the ART repertoire; the egg and sperm are combined in the laboratory, incubated, and the resulting embryos are transferred into the woman's uterus. The acronym sometimes used for this procedure is IVF/ET or IVF/ER, indicating embryo transfer or replacement.
- GIFT (Gamete IntraFallopian Transfer) Transfer of a mixture of eggs and sperm into the fallopian tube, allowing fertilization to take place within the fallopian tube.
- ZIFT (Zygote IntraFallopian Transfer) A combination of IVF and GIFT where fertilization takes place in vitro, but the resulting fertilized eggs (zygotes) are placed in the fallopian tube.
- PROST (Pronuclear Stage Tubal Transfer) A specific variation of ZIFT, but in this technique the embryo is in the pronuclear stage when it is transferred to the fallopian tube.
- TE(S)T (Tubal Embryo [Stage] Transfer) Another variation of ZIFT, in which an early divided embryo is transferred into the tube.

As you may have already realized, many of these procedures are very similar and some procedures, as defined by certain groups, may overlap. In some cases both GIFT and IVF are done, with transfer of eggs and sperm into the tube and embryos into the uterus.

3. Who is a candidate for ART? By the time you are ready to even approach consideration of these techniques, chances are that you will already have been through years of evaluation and treatment. In fact, one of our most important principles is that all the safer, simpler, and less expensive treatments should be considered before thinking of going on to the ART procedures.

Couples who have been through all the proper diagnostic tests and adequate trials of conventional treatment may be considered for the ART procedures if:

- The woman has tubal disease which has not been or cannot be overcome by surgery
- The man has a problem which has not been or cannot be treated by conventional measures
- The couple has a problem or problems which have not responded to conservative treatment
- The couple has no apparent cause for their inability to achieve a pregnancy and adequate time has been spent in conventional therapies.
- The couple is being evaluated and an ART procedure is being done in conjunction with that evaluation.

4. How successful are IVF and GIFT? Although the success rates of these procedures are improving, it is very important for you to have a realistic expectation of the chance of success. In fact, that's exactly what Dr. J. Benjamin Younger, president of The American Fertility Society (AFS), said in testimony before the House of Representatives Subcommittee on Regulation and Small Business Opportunities, the subcommittee that released the March 1989 survey of IVF/GIFT programs reported in Appendix 1.

The congressional survey, which was developed in conjunction with the American Fertility Society (AFS) and its affiliate Society for Assisted Reproductive Technology (SART), revealed that in 1987 the IVF "take-home" baby rate was 11.6 percent per egg retrieval procedure and 13.3 percent per embryo transfer. The clinical pregnancy rates are 16 percent for IVF and 25 percent for GIFT. As explained in Appendix 1, the 1988 data suffer from some significant errors but are probably somewhat higher than in 1987.

5. Do all IVF programs have similar results? The quoting of average figures obscures the most important finding in the survey— vast differences in success from one clinic to another, from a low of 0 percent to a high of 25 percent (in programs large enough to have significant experience). During 1988, there were over 16,000 IVF and/or GIFT procedures performed in the United States by the 96 clinics reporting to the AFS registry. The "take home" baby rates were 12 and 21 percent for IVF and GIFT respectively per egg retrieval and 3,427 babies were born.

These statistics may not sound too encouraging on the surface. But, as we have indicated previously and as Dr. Younger pointed out before the congressional committee, "a reproductively normal couple has [only] about a 20 percent chance of delivering a baby as a result of a single month's attempt and IVF patients are not reproductively normal." When you take that into account and add to that the fact that most of these couples were hopelessly infertile before this technology, those 1858 babies take on new meaning.

6. What sort of doctor am I looking for? Your first determination will be to decide what type of doctor or program you need. To a great extent, this will depend on where you are in the process of investigating your fertility problem. If you have never consulted a physician for your problem or have not had many tests, your own gynecologist is usually well equipped to handle the problem at this level and is probably the best place to begin.

If you have already been through the basic testing and have tried various treatments, it may be time to move on. Now you may want to seek a more specialized level of care, a physician who has had special training in reproductive medicine. He or she will be certified or a candidate for certification by the American Board of Obstetrics and Gynecology in the specialized area of reproductive endocrinology. These specialists can be found in individual practice, medical groups, fertility centers, and as directors of IVF programs.

7. If not all physicians are "created equal," how can we select the best one for us? Here's a breakdown of the major referral sources as we rank them from best to worst, according to objectivity and to the extent that each is mindful of your individual needs:

1. Physician or health professional who is a friend
2. Your own physician
3. Support groups (RESOLVE, Inc.)
4. Friend who has had good results
5. Prestigious hospital referral service
6. County medical society
7. Classified telephone directory

8. Once I have several names, how do I check to see which one is best for me? You have to do some investigation by calling or visiting the center to find out the answers to key questions. The first question usually relates to success rate. When that is answered to your satisfaction, other areas of concern will include how many cycles they do a year, the number of live births, and then the cost. Although all of these are good straightforward questions, the answers from some centers may not always be forthright.

9. How can I, as a layperson, evaluate their quoted success rate? We can never guarantee that the answers to your questions will be honest, but we feel that most centers will answer direct questions honestly. You just have to know the right questions.

First you must understand that pregnancy rates among programs are highly variable, with a number of teams having little or no success. Therefore, obtain a definite figure for success of the program you are investigating. Do not accept "average" success rates for *other* programs or for IVF as a whole. Average success rates for other programs have *no* relationship to the success rate of the particular program you are investigating.

It is important for you to understand how success rates are calculated because there can be a wide variation in rates based on a program's experience just by using different figures in the numerator and denominator.

10. Which rate is the best indicator of our chance to have a baby? In order to define the success rate you have to create a fraction. Ideally, the delivery rate of living babies is the most important numerator. This is because the definition of clinical pregnancy may vary among IVF programs, the level of miscarriage may be higher with poorer technique, and a live baby is really what you are striving for. But using the "live baby rate" is somewhat impractical since the rate of miscarriage may vary widely due to chance and there is an inherent nine-month delay from embryo transfer to delivery. Only well-established IVF programs can give a reasonably accurate "take-home baby rate." In addition, by the time you obtain a rate based on "take-home" babies, it is based on techniques used by personnel present over a year ago, a lengthy interval of time when considering ART procedures.

In the denominator we suggest egg retrievals rather than embryo transfer rate as the best reflection of IVF program quality because cases not reaching transfer could reflect deficiencies in egg retrieval or laboratory techniques and may give a falsely high success rate. The rate of cycle cancellation should also be examined because the success rate can be substantially influenced by allowing egg retrievals only when the results of stimulation are ideal. This rate is usually less than 20 percent. For practical purposes we suggest:

$$\frac{\text{CLINICAL PREGNANCIES}}{\text{EGG RETRIEVALS}} = \text{SUCCESS RATE}$$

Using this formula, you can use the figure of 10 percent clinical pregnancy rate per egg retrieval as the minimum level of performance to warrant confidence in an IVF program. Maximum rates have varied up to as high as 30 percent or more. For GIFT procedures, we would consider 15 percent a minimum to consider. Keep in mind, you are looking for excellence.

11. I have noticed that some of the very small programs have pretty good success rates. Should I consider a small program? We don't feel that you should necessarily shy away from very small programs. On the contrary, many are excellent and afford you the individualization you may desire. But, because of substantial variation based on chance alone, at least 100 cases are required to be able to quote a success rate that is a reasonably accurate reflection of the quality of the program. The variation based on chance alone, the inherent fertility potential of the couples happening to come through during a particular time, is enormous and vastly underestimated.

For example, in our program at AMI-South Bay Hospital we have had streaks of up to seven successful IVF cycles in a row. Consequently, we also have to experience occasional "dry spells." Because of this, we always recommend that you consider the success rate based on the last twelve months' experience rather than hearing that in the last month they had a streak of, for example, three pregnancies among twelve retrievals for a rate of 25 percent. They may not have had any pregnancies in the preceding two months.

12. How about a new program? Should I wait until they have some experience? Not necessarily. If a program has not been established for at least several years, inquire about how they learned these procedures. In order to learn the fine details that have proved successful through years of experience, these individuals must have prolonged and extensive experience with an established, successful program. If the individuals have a record they can quote with another program, the clinic may be worth considering although it is fairly new.

Keep in mind that just because a program has been established for several years does not mean that the same people who achieved the results reported are still working there. Ask: "How long has the team been together? Are the current members of the team the same people whose success rate they are quoting?" There is some tendency for personnel in this sophisticated field to move from program to program. This is a complex process requiring a team composed of individuals with training and experience in pelvic surgery, reproductive endocrinology, andrology, and embryology. The absence of one of these key people could have a devastating effect on an otherwise excellent program. There are instances of previously excellent programs that have no experienced people currently working on the team.

13. What if the program we are considering did not participate in the congressional survey? Some fine IVF and GIFT programs chose not to report to the congressional survey. Some of these programs do report to the Society for Assisted Reproductive Technology (SART), a specialty group of the American Fertility Society (AFS). We do not know why they didn't participate in the congressional survey. But it does not automatically mean that their success rates are not good. If you come across a program which did not participate, ask some hard-nosed questions about their lack of participation. If they report to SART, at least you have the reassurance that they are reporting their results, although SART has no power to alter or restrict their practices. If they are members of SART, you have the additional reassurance that they have, at least, met certain *minimal* criteria. Those criteria are a minimum of forty completed cycles per year as the qualifying level of activity to participate as a member. Additionally, the team must have experienced individuals at every level and must have had at least three live births from the program. Membership in SART assures you a minimum level of expertise and level of activity. There is, however, no assurance of a reasonable success rate since achieving a certain rate is not a requirement for membership.

14. We noticed a great deal of variation in the cost of IVF and GIFT among the centers we surveyed. How important is cost in making a decision? Only you can answer this question. Relative costs do vary quite a bit. As determined by the congressional panel, the cost of an IVF cycle runs some $4000 to $7000 for each attempt. The largest variable in determining cost will probably be geography, although centers in the same city may vary significantly. We certainly do *not* suggest that you "shop around" for the lowest price, but that you fit cost into the equation relative to its importance to you. Do not compromise quality for cost, but if two of the programs you are considering are similar, cost may become the deciding factor.

15. How do we decide whether to have IVF, GIFT, ZIFT, PROST, or TE(S)T? If your tubes are blocked, the choice is easy. IVF is the only appropriate method for you. If your problem is unrelated to a tubal factor, you have a choice. GIFT and the other procedures that utilize the fallopian tube for supporting gametes and embryos arose out of the frustration with low rates of success with IVF. Unless the IVF laboratory is functioning at a very high level, the fallopian tube is actually a better environment for the nourishment and growth of these cells. It is clearly evident, for example, that the transfer of eggs and sperm to the tube is more successful than IVF for the average U.S. program, since the rate of ongoing pregnancy with GIFT exceeded that with IVF by about 7 percent in 1986, 3 percent in 1987, and 9 percent in 1988. However, for many programs their individual rates for IVF approached or exceeded the national average for GIFT, suggesting that high-quality IVF approaches the results with GIFT.

The major procedural difference between IVF and GIFT is the need for laparoscopy for the latter as well as a major form of anesthesia. For many women who have had prior surgeries and anesthesia, the prospect of a procedure without incisions and under local anesthesia is enough to offset any small increase of pregnancy with GIFT. On the other hand, laparoscopy adds significant diagnostic aspects and the possibility of treatment for some women. Endometriosis may be evaluated and cauterized or vaporized and the status of the tubes and adhesions can be assessed.

One further difference between IVF and GIFT is the risk of tubal pregnancy. Although surveys have shown virtually equal rates (about 5 percent of pregnancies), tubal pregnancies with IVF occur almost exclusively in women with abnormal tubes, whereas most women undergoing GIFT have normal tubes. Therefore, in the women for whom either GIFT or IVF is appropriate, there is probably a small increase in the risk of ectopic pregnancy with GIFT. In women with tubal disease, the risk of ectopic with GIFT varies from 5 percent to 17 percent, depending upon the extent of the tubal damage.

Then what about ZIFT/PROST/TE(S)T? It is not clear whether ZIFT/ PROST/TE(S)T carries a higher rate of pregnancy than GIFT. Therefore it may be considered when a male factor or the presence of antisperm antibodies may impair fertilization with GIFT. Fertilization is more certain, as with IVF, and the placement of embryos into the tubes allows a further one to two days of development in the normal location and a normal entry into the uterus. However, it requires *both* transvaginal egg retrieval and laparoscopy, with accompanying increased discomfort and expense. The increased pregnancy rate is likely to be proportional to the increased cost, but a patient might prefer to save those financial resources for an additional IVF cycle and avoid the increased discomfort of an operative procedure.

You can see that the choice of ART procedure is not easy and depends upon the success rate achieved with IVF in a particular program, the potential for diagnostic information, and the patient's outlook toward surgery, anesthesia, and tubal pregnancy.

16. What if the program I am considering does only one of these procedures? We feel that in 1990 a quality program should have *all* the current methods of treatment available. An example might be embryo freezing. Except when a woman is older or embryo quality is reduced, limiting the number of fresh embryos transferred to three or four can better control the risk of multiple pregnancy. Freezing additional embryos can reduce costs considerably by allowing multiple embryo transfer procedures from one stimulation and retrieval. In some women, the uterus may not be receptive in the stimulated cycle. So, if embryo freezing is not available in a particular program, you may be limiting your chances for success.

17. What actually is involved in an IVF cycle? Before a patient is placed in the program, we feel that all other conventional treatments should be exhausted. This may include cycles with stimulation of multiple ovulation with Pergonal associated with intrauterine insemination in patients with open tubes. Certain tests should be done if they have not been performed recently. We recommend a current semen analysis, test for sperm antibodies in the husband and wife, sperm penetration assay, chlamydia culture or antibiotic treatment, and a "trial transfer." We believe that the transfer is the most critical part of the process and that a rehearsal of this process with a mapping of the cervical canal is most useful.

The procedure of in vitro fertilization/embryo transfer itself consists of four basic steps, all of which will be accomplished within the time frame of one menstrual cycle and will take approximately thirty days:

1. Ripening of the egg(s)
2. Retrieval of the eggs
3. Fertilization of the eggs and growth of the resulting embryos
4. Transfer of the embryo(s) into the uterus (ET)

18. Do I need surgery to have the eggs retrieved? At this time almost everyone is using transvaginal ultrasound guided egg retrieval. However, there are still some holdouts for laparoscopy. The ultrasound technique, described elsewhere in the book, utilizes sedation rather than anesthesia and requires less recovery time. Patients who have experienced both uniformly prefer the ultrasound technique. The only drawback to ultrasound aspiration is that the diagnostic and therapeutic aspects of laparoscopy are lost. In some individual cases there may be aspects important enough to justify the additional expense and risk of laparoscopy. Of course, with GIFT and ZIFT, laparoscopy is required.

19. Is there an age limit for ART procedures? We generally limit these procedures to couples in which the woman has not reached her forty-second birthday. In cases in which donor eggs are being used, we accept women up to forty-six. On a practical basis, the limit of forty-two for the use of one's own eggs is because the success rates are poor over age forty-two, with a term birth rate of less than 5 percent currently being achieved, even in very good programs.

20. Is IVF a stressful procedure? It is a very intense and stressful procedure for the couple. For this reason, we feel that an experienced program should have readily available psychological support to optimize the couple's ability to cope with the stresses inherent in the process. Psychological issues can have a major impact on the success of an individual couple, since perseverence is a key to the ultimate chance of a pregnancy. Emotional stability and mutual support help a couple persist in their quest. And as we have said repeatedly, *persistence is the key to success!*

Remember, the answers to these twenty questions will provide you with only a quick introduction to the subject of assisted reproduction. Be a good consumer. Learn all you can before making a decision. Choosing a quality program will have a significant influence on your chances for having a baby. Good luck!

GLOSSARY

AATB   American Association of Tissue Banks
adhesions   scar tissue
AFS   American Fertility Society
agonist   compound that is almost identical chemically with another but may have the opposite effect metabolically
amniocentesis   withdrawal of a sample of fluid contained in the pregnancy sac
amenorrhea   lack of menstrual period
andrologist   specialist in male reproductive function
anovulation   lack of ovulation
antisperm antibodies   proteins that can specifically attach to sperm, impairing their function
ART   assisted reproductive technology
aspiration (follicle)   withdrawal of fluid surrounding the egg
assisted reproductive technology (ART)   technical manipulation of the sperm and egg outside the body for replacement into the reproductive organs to achieve a pregnancy
asthenospermia   poor movement of sperm
azoospermia   the complete absence of sperm in the ejaculate
basal body temperature (BBT)   body temperature upon awakening, before any activity
BBT   basal body temperature
beta HCG   the specific part of the pregnancy hormone that is measured to diagnose pregnancy
biochemical pregnancy   a positive blood test for HCG but without ultrasound evidence of pregnancy or miscarriage less than four weeks after embryo transfer

bromocriptine (Parlodel)   drug used to reduce elevated levels of prolactin in treating galactorreha, amenorrhea, and prolactin-secreting tumors of the pituitary

capacitation   development of the ability of sperm to fertilize an egg

cervical mucus   mucus produced by the cervix that thins before ovulation to assist sperm migration

cervix   the opening of the uterus

chlamydia   an organism, generally sexually transmitted, that can cause tubal damage

chromosomes   tiny collections of genetic material within a cell nucleus

clinical pregnancy   evidence of pregnancy by ultrasound, passage of pregnancy tissue in a miscarriage, or delivery of a fetus or baby

Clomid   brand name of clomiphene citrate

clomiphene citrate (Serophene, Clomid)   an oral medication that stimulates ovulation

conceptus   the developing zygote, pre-embryo, or embryo resulting from the joining of the sperm and egg

corpus luteum   hormone producing tissue in the ovary that develops from the collapsed follicle, produces hormones, and supports early pregnancy

cryopreservation   deep-freezing by techniques that allow survival and growth of cells after thawing

cumulative pregnancy rate   the chance of a couple conceiving over a period of time

cumulus cells   the expanded clear mucus-like tissue surrounding the egg

danazol (Danocrine)   drug used to treat endometriosis

Danocrine   brand name of danazol

DES   diethylstilbestrol

diethylstilbestrol   a synthetic estrogen, given to women in the 1950s, 1960s, and early 1970s, to prevent miscarriage, that resulted in abnormalities of the reproductive tract of female offspring

ectopic pregnancy   growth of a pregnancy in any location other than the uterine cavity, known commonly as tubal pregnancy

egg retrieval   aspiration of eggs from the ovary

ejaculate   the sperm and glandular fluid released when a man reaches sexual climax (ejaculation)

embryo   the result of the fertilization of the egg by the sperm; the developing individual from conception to the end of the second month

embryo transfer (replacement)   placement of embryos into the reproductive tract

embryologist   a person trained to work with gametes and embryos

endometrial biopsy   sample of tissue obtained from the endometrium to assess its maturity and ability to promote implantation of the embryo

endometrioma   a cyst within the ovary caused by endometriosis and containing a dark-brown chocolatelike fluid

endometriosis   a disease in which endometrium grows outside the uterus

endometrium   the tissue lining the cavity of the uterus

epididymis   part of tubular system where sperm collect after leaving the testicles

estradiol   the principal active estrogen in women

estrogen   a hormone that has stimulating effects on the uterus and breasts

ER (embryo replacement)   placement of an embryo into the reproductive tract

ET (embryo transfer)   embryo replacement

fallopian tube   a reproductive structure, a thin tubal structure that picks up the egg from the ovary, supports fertilization and early embryo development, and transports the embryo to the uterus

fertilization   union of the sperm and egg resulting in the development of the zygote

fibroid   benign muscle tumor of the wall of the uterus

follicle   fluid-filled space and surrounding tissue that envelop the egg

follicle-stimulating hormone (FSH)   hormone that stimulates growth of the follicle

fimbria   delicate fingerlike tissue at the end of the fallopian tube that picks up the egg from the ovary

FSH (Metrodin)   follicle-stimulating hormone

galactorrhea   milklike discharge from the breasts

gamete   reproductive cells; sperm in the male, ova in the female

gamete intrafallopian transfer (GIFT)   placement of sperm and eggs into the fallopian tube

germ cells   sperm and egg

GIFT   gamete intrafallopian transfer

GnRH   gonadotropin releasing hormone

GnRH analogue   compound that is almost identical chemically with GnRH but can have the opposite metabolic action

gonadotropin-releasing hormone   a hormone that stimulates the pituitary to release FSH and LH

gonadotropins   the hormones FSH and LH, which act on the ovary to control its function

gonads   reproductive organs that produce gametes and hormones; the testicles and ovaries

HCG   human chorionic gonadotropin

health maintenance organization (HMO)   a form of health insurance where the premium prepays all expenses and providers are strictly limited to those within the plan. Generally no reimbursement is provided for physicians outside the health plan unless prior arrangements are made, with the plan making the referral.

hMG (Pergonal)   human menopausal gonadotropin

HMO   health maintenance organization

human chorionic gonadotropin (HCG)   hormone produced by the conceptus and later the placenta that can be measured to diagnose pregnancy

human menopausal gonadotropin (hMG; Pergonal)   preparation of FSH and LH derived from menopausal urine

hydrosalpinx   dilated fluid-filled, obstructed fallopian tube
hypothalamus   area of the brain just above the pituitary gland that controls many hormone-producing glands through its effects on the pituitary
hysterosalpingogram   X-ray of the inside of the uterus ~d tubes; employs a radio-opaque dye
hysteroscopy   examination of the inside of the uterus using a telescope placed through the cervix
infertility   generally, the inability of a couple to conceive within one year
intrauterine device (IUD)   device worn inside the uterine cavity to prevent pregnancy
intrauterine insemination (IUI)   placement of sperm, usually washed, into the uterine cavity
in vitro fertilization (IVF)   most advanced procedure in the ART repertoire: the sperm and egg are combined in the laboratory, incubated, and the resulting embryos are transferred into the woman's uterus; literally, fertilization "in glass"
IUD   intrauterine device
IUI   intrauterine insemination
IVF   in vitro fertilization
IVF/ER   in vitro fertilization/embryo replacement
IVF/ET   in vitro fertilization/embryo transfer
laparoscopy   examination of the abdomen and pelvic organs by means of a telescope placed through an incision in the navel
LH   luteinizing hormone
LH surge   marked increase of release of LH into the blood, which causes final maturation of the egg and its release from the follicle
liquification   process by which semen changes consistency from jellylike to liquid
LPD   luteal-phase defect
LUF   luteinized unruptured follicle
Lupron (leuprolide)   medication similar to GnRH, used to suppress the pituitary and, in turn, the ovaries
luteal phase   phase of the menstrual cycle from ovulation until menses
luteal-phase defect (LPD)   poor development of the endometrium in preparation for implantation
luteinized unruptured follicle (LUF)   failure of the follicle to rupture and release the egg
luteinizing hormone   a hormone released from the pituitary that causes ovulation and stimulates the corpus luteum to secrete progesterone
male factor   a term for infertility originating in the male partner
Metrodin   brand name of pure FSH
microsurgery   surgery using fine instruments, magnification, and gentle handling of the tissues, usually on the fallopian tubes
monthly conception rate   the chance of a couple conceiving within the woman's one-month cycle
morphology   categorization of sperm by their shape
motility   the percentage of sperm moving in a sample of semen

mycoplasma   an organism that can colonize the reproductive tract and damage the tubes or cause miscarriage

oocytes   eggs

ovary   female reproductive organ that produces eggs and hormones

ovulation   release of an egg from the follicle

PCO   polycystic ovarian disease

PCT   post coital test

pelvic adhesions   scar-tissue band capable of covering or distorting organs; most commonly affect fallopian tubes, ovaries, and bowel

pelvic inflammatory disease (PID)   a general term for pelvic infections resulting from sexually transmitted diseases.

pelviscopy   synonym for laparoscopy, although often used to indicate operative laparoscopy

Pergonal   brand of human menopausal gonadotropin (hMG)

PID   pelvic inflammatory disease

pituitary   a hormone-producing gland lying under the base of the brain that controls the function of the adrenals, thyroid, ovaries, and testicles

polycystic ovarian disease (PCO)   condition characterized by hormonal imbalance and lack of ovulation

polyspermia   fertilization of the egg by more than one sperm

post coital test (PCT)   a test of the cervical mucus after intercourse

PPO (preferred provider organization)   a form of health insurance where the insurance company makes contractual arrangements with "preferred providers" for better rates. The patient is not required to go to a specific provider but will generally get better coverage through a preferred provider—for example, 80 percent reimbursement rather than 50 percent through a nonpreferred entity.

premature ovarian failure   cessation of normal ovarian function before the usual age of menopause, generally before forty

progesterone   hormone that causes the endometrium to develop changes to make it receptive to the embryo

progestin   synthetic hormone with action similar to progesterone

prolactin   hormone released from the pituitary that causes the breasts to secrete milk

pronuclear stage transfer (PROST)   transfer of the conceptus at or shortly after the pronuclear stage.

pronucleus (ei)   the male and female nuclei that are visible 14–18 hours after combining sperm with an egg

PROST   pronuclear stage transfer

RESOLVE, Inc.   a nonprofit organization helping people with infertility by offering counseling, medical referral, emotional support, and literature as well as education and assistance to associated professionals

retrograde ejaculation   passage of semen back into the bladder during ejaculation

retrograde menstrual flow   flow of menses back through the fallopian tubes into the pelvic cavity

salpingitis   inflammation (infection) of the fallopian tubes

salpingostomy   incision into the fallopian tube

SART   Society for Assisted Reproductive Technology

selective termination   a procedure that aborts one or more fetuses of a multiple pregnancy, usually quadruplets or more

semen   the combination of sperm and glandular fluid released from the penis when a man reaches sexual climax

seminal vesicles   glands that add fluid to the semen to assist sperm deposition

Serophene   brand name of clomiphene citrate

sexually transmitted disease (STD)   diseases caused by organisms that are transmitted by sexual contact and activity

SPA   sperm penetration assay

sperm penetration assay (SPA)   test of fertilizing capacity of the sperm using zona-free hamster eggs

STD   sexually transmitted disease

Stein–Leventhal Syndrome   early term for a severe form of polycystic ovarian disease (PCO)

subfertility   synonym for infertility implying that the ability to conceive is less than normal

ultrasound   high frequency sound waves used to make an image of body structures

ureaplasma   type of mycoplasma implicated in male infertility and miscarriage

TE(S)T   tubal embryo (stage) transfer

testicle   male sex organ that produces sperm and hormones

tubal embryo (stage) transfer [TE(S)T]   transfer of dividing embryos into the fallopian tube

urethra   the urinating channel leading from the bladder to the outside through the penis

uterus   the womb; a muscular organ that carries the developing fetus

vagina   a tubular structure leading from the vulva to the cervix

varicocele   dilation of the spermatic veins that causes a backflow of blood to the testes and impaired sperm function

varicocelectomy   operation for repair of varicocele

vas deferens   muscular tube that carries sperm from the epididymis to the urethra

vasovasostomy   operation for reversal of male sterilization (vasectomy)

viscosity   the thickness of the semen, evaluated after a period of time following ejaculation

ZIFT   zygote intrafallopian transfer

zona drilling   the making of a hole in the shell (zona) that surrounds the egg

zona pellucida   the shell that surrounds the egg and protects it during early embryo development

zygote   fertilized egg

zygote intrafallopian transfer (ZIFT)   transfer of fertilized egg(s) to the fallopian tube

Index